YOUR BODY, YOUR CHOICE

SHANNON FARMER & DAVID WEBB

MEDIA MASTERS

SINGAPORE

Your Body, Your Choice
Copyright © 2000 by Shannon Farmer, David Webb
and Media Masters Pte Ltd

Published by: Media Masters Pte Ltd,
Newton Road PO Box 272, Singapore 912210.
Email: medmas@mbox3.singnet.com.sg
Website: www.mediamasters.com.sg
Fax: (65) 484-2559

Editing and photography: Media Masters Pte Ltd
Design: Wendy Wong
Printed by Mui Kee Press & Co. Singapore.

First published August 2000

Note to readers:
Your Body, Your Choice covers many aspects of blood, including its history in the medical context and associated subjects. It provides up-to-date information about medical and surgical management alternatives to allogeneic blood transfusion (bloodless medicine and surgery). As indicated by the lengthy bibliography and other references, every effort was made to ensure accuracy at time of printing on a subject which is undergoing constant review and research. The manuscript was also reviewed by a number of internationally eminent physicians. The contents of this book are provided for information only. Such information does not constitute medical advice and should not be relied upon as such. Under no circumstances does **Your Body, Your Choice** recommend particular treatment for specific individuals. In all cases, the authors advise that a physician be consulted before any course of treatment is pursued. References in the book to particular drugs, treatment or procedures do not constitute either their endorsement or their recommended use.

ISBN: 981-04-1708-X

PREFACE

Your Body, Your Choice is about the ground-breaking impact of bloodless medicine and surgery – medical and surgical treatment without blood transfusion. It is the first book published for the general reader on the most significant, yet largely unheralded, advances being made in modern medical practice.

In lay person's language, the authors identify why and how bloodless surgery is set to become standard practice at hospitals and medical centers worldwide. They explain the make-up of blood, how it works and its role in medical history. They relate how past acceptance of blood transfusion and its presumed benefits are now being questioned against increasing recognition that blood, the lifesaver, has also become blood, the killer.

Medical opinion is gradually turning full circle since the rapid expansion of donor blood banks at the end of the Second World War. The profession is seeing a paradigm shift in transfusion practice, tragically underwritten by major catastrophes in which thousands of people died after being given infected blood. Subsequent medical discoveries concerning the effects of transfused blood on the immune system and on the ability of the body to recover quickly have also helped encourage a safer new approach to treatment. Where bloodless surgery was once the small domain of specialized institutions and dedicated individuals serving the interests of those who refused transfusions for religious reasons, it is now practiced to a degree in most developed countries. Given the advances taking place in technology and science, some experts are predicting blood transfusion will be obsolete within 10 to 15 years.

Ironically, against this rapidly changing background, most people are generally unaware of bloodless surgery and the profound impact it is likely to have on their lives. Similarly, many doctors are not fully acquainted with the progress being made in this area of medicine. Moreover, they choose to stay with the practices in which they were trained. Sadly, in these circumstances, the natural human resistance to change is putting lives at risk.

Your Body, Your Choice is not only the first book of its kind on the subject for the lay person; it is also, as eminent reviewers agree, a book destined to be a valuable reference for medical practitioners.

CONTENTS

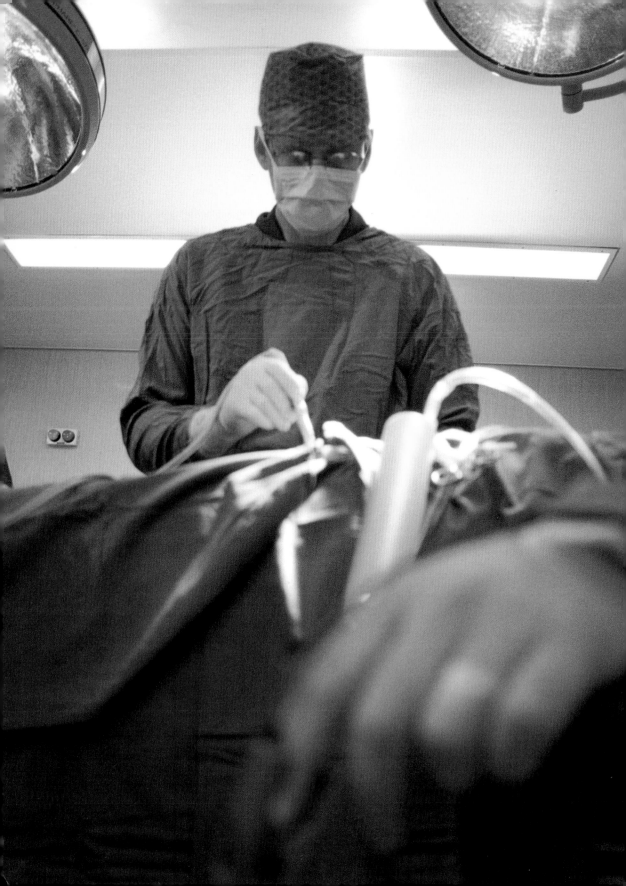

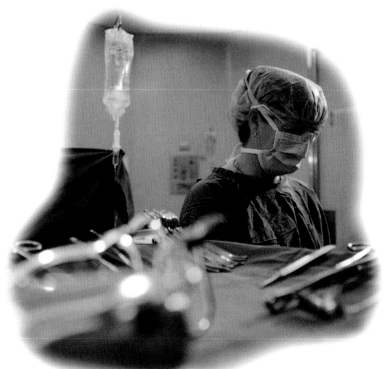

CHAPTER 1

WHY SURGERY WITHOUT BLOOD?

Chapter

Liver Transplant: a Case History

*I*n the mid-1990s, a young Californian man was admitted to hospital in a very serious state brought on by acute liver failure. In addition to other symptoms, he had encephalopathy, a serious disorder of the brain and nervous system. He was days – possibly hours – away from death. The documented account of the 23-year-old patient was reported in the 1996 issue of the medical journal *Clinical Transplantation*. While the patient's identity must be protected in line with that report, we shall call him William for the purposes of this account.

Two weeks before being taken to hospital, William had been his normal, healthy self. Then he developed symptoms of nausea, vomiting and weakness in his limbs. He rapidly became jaundiced and mentally confused. He also suffered gastro-intestinal bleeding. William's condition had deteriorated so much that doctors immediately placed him on an artificial breathing machine. They assessed his survival depended on an urgent liver transplant.

The operation William required was one of the most difficult, challenging and bloody procedures faced by surgeons. The liver controls more than 500 chemical reactions. Among its functions, it manufactures a number of plasma proteins, clotting factors and bile salts for digestion. It collects and stores nutrients and filters out many of the body's toxins, converting some to less dangerous products. But when a person goes into liver failure, toxins bypass the normal filtering system and end up in the brain and nervous system. The effects are fast and devastating. Patients can slip quickly from being confused to psychotic. They can suffer seizures and lapse into unconsciousness. In the most severe cases, irreversible coma and death follow.

In the past, liver transplants had required an average of 43 units of transfused whole blood or red blood cells. In some cases as many as 300 units were used.[1] Although advancing techniques and experience had reduced blood loss considerably, the majority of surgeons as recently as the late 1980s still believed liver transplantation to be impossible without blood transfusion, even in the best circumstances.

But by the mid-1990s, at the time of William's illness, the picture was changing. Public awareness of the growing list of potential and inherent risks and hazards associated with receiving another person's blood had created a mushrooming interest in alternatives to blood transfusion. William was one of a growing number of people who, for personal or medical reasons, were now refusing the option of transfused blood.

Consequently, the young man's refusal, coupled with his critically advanced condition, presented medical staff with an enormous dilemma. The hospital concluded it far too hazardous to attempt an operation without donor blood. With options fast diminishing, doctors decided to treat him with support medication. It amounted to a desperate effort to address his symptoms.

The medication, however, had little effect. As the patient's condition continued to deteriorate, the hospital contacted a transplant center in California which agreed to carry out the operation without a transfusion. By the time William was transferred to the center he was in a coma. He had lost a significant amount of blood from internal bleeding. Moreover, there was a further serious complication. As his liver had failed, his blood-clotting factors were very low. In other words, William's blood was extremely "thin" and this, in turn, placed him at serious risk of a life-threatening hemorrhage during surgery.

In the face of intensifying complications, the medical team had little choice but to proceed urgently with the liver transplant. Time was of the essence. The team recognized they were about to undertake one of the most demanding of operations. A surgical procedure of this nature without resort to transfused blood on a man whose life was so delicately balanced would be the ultimate test of their knowledge and skills.

Fortunately for William, a donor became available within hours. The medical team went to work. By the time the operation was over, William had lost less than two cupfuls of blood and received no blood transfusion. This, compared with the earlier average of 43 units! Seven days after the procedure, he was wheeled from intensive care to a general ward. He spent a further 11 days in hospital and was discharged just 19 days after he was first admitted in a life-threatening, comatose state. Six months later, William was reported doing well, his blood count back to normal.

In the same year that William's case was reported, on the other side of the Atlantic the first liver transplantation without blood transfusion was carried out successfully on a 47-year-old woman who had refused blood because of her religious beliefs.

A medical team (pictured right) at St James's University Hospital in Leeds operated on Mrs Linda Pearson, a mother of four, who suffered from primary biliary cirrhosis of the liver, an auto-immune condition that was destroying her liver. Without a transplant, she had been told, she would have only three years to live.

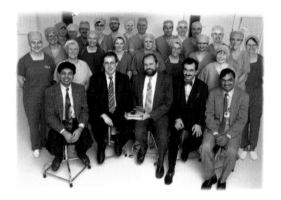

To go ahead with such an operation would, normally, have meant transfusing multiple units of blood. In her circumstances, however, transfusion was out of the question. After weeks of discussion with her surgeon, Stephen Pollard, and anaesthetist Dr Mark Bellamy, a protocol was decided on. Mr Pollard, who is director of the liver and intestinal transplant unit at St James's, said in a subsequent newspaper report: "We gave her an absolute undertaking that even if her life was under threat, we would not give her blood."

In the lead-up to the operation, Mrs Pearson injected herself daily with the hormone erythropoietin to boost the production of oxygen-carrying red blood cells (see Chapter 5). On the day of the operation, Mr Pollard operated slowly, keeping incisions small and not proceeding before any cut blood vessel was tied.

The operation was a complete success. A year later, Mrs Pearson was again leading a normal life and was able to tell an interviewer: "It was teamwork. The doctors said I took the risks, but I think that they did. I wanted to live and I was appealing to their expertise. I knew I might not survive but I had great confidence in the doctors."

Other "bloodless" procedures have since been successfully carried out by the St James's Hospital medical team. More recently, 19-year-old computer science student Ewan Opperman flew from South Africa to Leeds for liver transplantation after surgeons in Cape Town would not carry out a similar operation. Within four weeks, the patient was well enough to fly home.

Why Bloodless Surgery Makes Sense

As with William and Linda Pearson, many thousands of surgical operations are increasingly being carried out internationally without resort to allogeneic[2] blood transfusion.

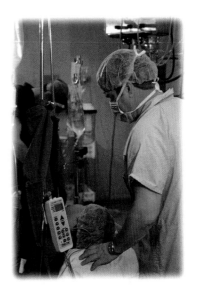

Surgery without blood transfusion has been practiced on a small scale since the 1950s. Those who initially sought treatment without transfusion did so primarily for religious reasons. Today, however, the growing list of diseases that can be carried in blood has caused a worldwide undercurrent of concern. The simple truth is there can be no guarantees. Donated blood, however meticulous the screening methods, remains a potential health threat.

Despite this, most people are unaware of bloodless surgery and how it may benefit them. Try introducing the subject of "bloodless surgery" to anyone and the first response is raised eyebrows and a quick dismissal. "Bloodless surgery, how can you have surgery without blood? It doesn't make sense."

To some the terminology is confusing. If you cut your hand, you bleed. So how can surgeons carry out major operations without causing bleeding?

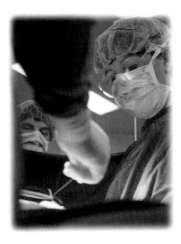

The answer is simple. They can't. Well, not quite — yet. By using appropriate *combinations* of medicines, surgical equipment and innovative techniques, surgeons can reduce bleeding to a point where there is relatively little blood loss. All of the drugs, devices and techniques employed this way are well known in medical science. Some have been improved, modified or combined with new technology. However, at the core of all the innovation lies the unwavering objective: to provide the best possible patient care using **medical and**

11

surgical treatment without allogeneic blood transfusion. Hence the name, bloodless medicine and surgery.[3]

As an official publication from the Good Samaritan Hospital in Los Angeles puts it: "Otherwise known as 'bloodless', transfusion-free medicine and surgery is a state-of-the-art approach to the proper management of a disease or condition. It employs both non-invasive medical care and invasive/surgical care as part of a strategy to avoid blood transfusion. Transfusion-free medicine and surgery incorporates the best, documented, rational approaches available, and should not be misunderstood as a less effective 'alternative therapy.' The techniques of transfusion-free medicine and surgery are a state-of-the-art synthesis of new and older approaches to medical and surgical care – the best care possible."

The case history of William, cited at the outset of this chapter, is a good example of how bloodless medicine and surgery can be carried out even in one of the most difficult of all surgical operations. The liver is very vascular. It gets two blood supplies. One comes from a network of veins which introduces blood full of nutrients from the digestive tract. The other flows through an artery, which feeds the organ with necessary oxygen. As one surgeon quipped: "You only have to look at the liver and it bleeds."

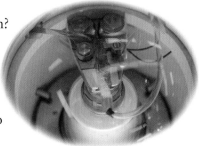

So what happened to William during the operation? The surgeon, the anesthesiologist and the operating room team combined a number of drugs, devices and techniques to reduce William's blood loss and maximize his ability to transport oxygen to his cells. A cell saver machine (pictured right) was also

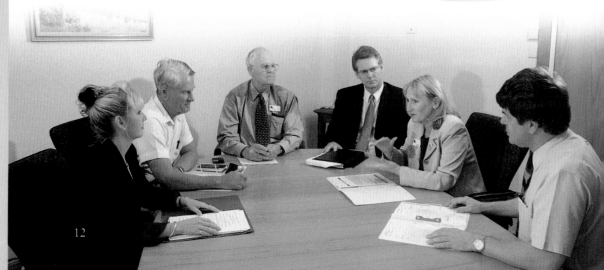

used to collect any blood lost during the operation and return it to his bloodstream.

After the operation, special nutrients and medications were given William to boost further his blood production and recovery. Later in the book, you will read detailed descriptions of these techniques.

"Gift of Life" . . . "Bringer of Death"

Until recently, it was generally accepted that to be given someone else's donated blood was the gift of life. However, there is growing international recognition that the traditional reliance on blood as a lifesaver is no longer fully supportable. Indeed, the tide of scientific and medical opinion in today's changing society opens to question the whole practice of blood transfusion. This was brought to the attention of the public dramatically in the 1980s with the realization that the deadly HIV/AIDS virus could be transmitted by blood.

As the years passed, public apprehension intensified. *Popular Science* magazine, in its June 1993 edition, made the observation: "Fear has become a dominating factor in the world of blood transfusions with AIDS the greatest driving force behind the fear." What the public had perceived as the gift of life now was seen to have the potential of bringing death.

The possibility of contracting a virus or disease from contaminated blood is not the only reason why more and more people are looking for safer alternatives. In 1987, Dr Richard Walker, writing in the *American Journal of Clinical Pathology*, reported that about 20% of all transfusions resulted in some type of adverse effect. Three years later, Dr Charles Huggins, Director of Transfusion Services at the Massachusetts General Hospital, was quoted in the Boston Globe Magazine: "Blood has never been safer. But it must be considered unavoidably non-safe. It is the most dangerous substance we use in medicine."

Scientific research continues to make new discoveries about the very nature of blood itself and its frequent negative side-effects. For instance, it is now well documented that one person's blood transfused to another alters many facets of the recipient's immune system, leaving it more vulnerable to infection and disease. There is also mounting evidence that if blood is given at the time of cancer surgery, the cancer may recur sooner and survival time will be shortened. This underscores another major worry about transfusion: blood does not have to be contaminated for tragic sequels to occur.

On the other hand, bloodless surgery techniques not only reduce the risk of exposure to diseases, they also have a number of other tangible benefits for patients. For example, recovery from an operation is generally quicker for the bloodless surgery patient. This, of course, has very significant implications for the availability and cost of hospital resources. A Canadian hospital has reported that by reducing the use of transfused blood in liver transplantation, hospital stay-days decreased by almost half. This positive trend has been borne out time and again for a whole range of major procedures managed without allogeneic blood transfusion. The list now includes:

- Burns
- Obstetrics
- Cardiac surgery
- Orthopedic surgery
- Cancer surgery
- Pediatric surgery
- General surgery
- Plastic surgery
- Gynecological surgery
- Transplantation of organs
- Hematological disorders
- Trauma
- Neonatology
- Urological surgery
- Neurosurgery
- Vascular surgery

Early Days of Modern Bloodless Medicine and Surgery

The bloodless approach encompasses some of the most rapidly advancing areas of medicine today. However, it is also important to understand that bloodless surgery is not something that has emerged only recently as a result of viral epidemics. The spread of diseases like AIDS and hepatitis C are comparatively new cogs in the wheel that has been driving bloodless surgery since the 1950s.

American surgeon Denton Cooley (pictured) generally recognized as "the father of modern bloodless surgery," pioneered open-heart surgery without blood transfusion at the

14

Texas Heart Institute in 1957. Initially, his efforts were directed at treating patients who requested transfusion-free surgery for religious reasons. At that time, up to 12 units of blood were used just to prime the heart-lung machine. Operations themselves routinely required the transfusion of 20 to 30 units. Cooley and his team developed methods of priming the heart-lung machine with non-blood fluids which became known as "bloodless prime". As other techniques were developed to avoid the use of blood, they were referred to as "bloodless techniques". Thus the term "bloodless surgery" emerged.

Cooley had outstanding success. He reported on hundreds of bloodless surgery operations undertaken on children and adults — from one-day-olds to 89-year-olds — saying that such methods avoided the complications often experienced with transfusions. His good results led him to recommend these techniques be used more extensively.

In 1973, heart surgeon Jerome Kay, writing in *The Journal of the American Medical Association,* commented on similar good results: "We have now done approximately 6,000 open-heart operations at the Saint Vincent's Hospital in Los Angeles. Since we have not been using blood for the majority of patients, it is our impression that the patients do better."

Other specialists gradually embraced these techniques and applied them to abdominal, orthopedic, transplantation, urologic, cancer and other surgical fields with similar results.

Cooley's distinguished role was recognized in a 1995 issue of *The American Journal of Surgery* in which the editor-in-chief, Dr Hiram C. Polk Jr, praised the surgeon for the lead he had taken. He stated that before anyone else even contemplated doing so, Cooley performed open-heart surgery without blood transfusion on 1,250 patients who requested it for religious reasons. "Dr Cooley's blood conservation techniques," he wrote, "are applicable to every operation and, therefore, meaningful to all 17,000 readers of *The American Journal of Surgery.*" He went on to note that Cooley's "attention to detail to minimize blood loss should become a model for all surgical specialties." The article ended on an auspicious note: "Some of his operative tricks should be standard procedure for all of us."

The following year, Professor Jacques Belghiti told a bloodless surgery international symposium in Paris that in his opinion a good operation was one with no blood loss. To achieve this, surgeons needed to slow down, take their time, operate meticulously, carefully and smoothly, and not accept bleeding as inevitable. The challenge had prompted doctors to adopt increasingly sophisticated strategies including the use of ultrasound scalpels, microwave scalpels, argon beam coagulators and a variety of clamping techniques. Anesthesiologists had also risen to the challenge. They had developed blood-salvaging techniques and extended the limits of hemodilution. Professor Belghiti concluded: "I am convinced that what is considered a challenge today will be considered good medical practice tomorrow."

A significant new development occurred in the 1970s. A team of doctors, who had already played a pivotal role in pioneering the new "bloodless" approach, established The Institute of Bloodless Medicine and Surgery in California. The group was headed by surgeon Ron Lapin and anesthesiologist Fred Garcia. Lapin was a controversial surgeon whose skills in carrying out the most delicate procedures, often in high-risk circumstances, earned him worldwide recognition.

The California team brought together a coordinated, formal program specializing in all the disciplines of surgery without blood. By 1986, Lapin, Garcia and their team were able to report their experience with several thousand patients who had undergone major surgery and anesthesia without the use of blood or blood products. The operations had covered all surgical specialties, including general, brain, heart, chest, vascular, cancer, urinary tract, gynecology and orthopedic (joint replacement and spinal) surgery. Emergency operations had also been carried out successfully on patients who had hemorrhaged and lost up to 90% of their blood volume.

Rapid Growth of Centers

The California team's experience reaffirmed Cooley's earlier published findings where he stated his young patients "do as well or better" than those who had blood transfusions. The group also established that the mortality rate and incidence of morbidity (a diseased, abnormal or disordered condition) among their patients compared favorably with procedures where blood transfusions were used.

By this time, medical interest in bloodless surgery had spread beyond California across the nation. In 1987, the John F Kennedy Medical Center in Chicago

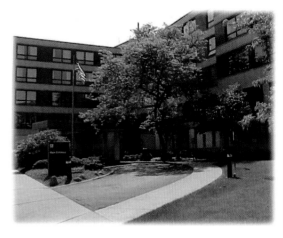

(soon after renamed Our Lady of the Resurrection Medical Center, pictured right), pioneered the new concept of a Center for Bloodless Medicine and Surgery within a larger hospital setting. A hospital-appointed taskforce set about assembling a team of doctors and other health care professionals, buying specialized equipment and developing the necessary protocols. More than 40 physicians joined the program. They willingly made themselves available at all times for consultation with other hospitals and accepted emergency patients transferred to them. The center's commitment to the principle of bloodless surgery established a highly successful program which soon became standard practice. Today the hospital treats a steady stream of patients from local areas, surrounding states and from as far away as Mississippi and Canada.

These were the very first efforts to establish units specializing in bloodless medicine and surgery. There are now more than 200 internationally, ranging from small community hospitals to large university teaching hospitals.

Emergency Cases

As the fledgling medical center in Chicago soon found out, there was an urgent need for the bloodless treatment of emergency patients. This has become increasingly evident with the growth of bloodless surgery. The following examples are typical.

A cardiothoracic (heart and chest) surgeon, with whom author Shannon Farmer has worked, was involved in the treatment of a car accident victim who had lost a massive amount of blood. He was an elderly man with coronary artery disease who had undergone bypass surgery some years earlier. In the accident he had sustained serious injuries including a ruptured aorta (the main large blood vessel coming out of the heart), a ruptured spleen and a ruptured diaphragm. He had also refused blood for religious reasons. His condition was so bad that, in the opinion of one doctor on duty, he would not survive the night without blood. Emergency surgery was performed during which bleeding was arrested through various techniques described in chapters 5 and 6. Following the operation, he was placed on a ventilator in the intensive care unit and given blood-building medications. The ventilator is a mechanical device delivering oxygen to the lungs under pressure. Other supportive measures (described later in the book) were used. He survived, despite being elderly, having heart problems and having bled down to a hemoglobin of 4 g/dL (grams per deciliter). Normal for an average adult male is 14 – 18 g/dL. The man went on to enjoy good quality of life for many years.

Another trauma case, with which Farmer was involved, concerned a 40-year-old man who had a horrific motor vehicle accident in 1996. He was driving his flat-nosed fruit van along a highway when a steel delivery truck pulled out directly in front of him from a side road. With no time to brake, he slammed head-on into the side of the truck. It took an hour to cut him from the wreckage. The man sustained many serious injuries, among them, fractures of the skull, nose, upper and lower jaw, ribs, shoulder blade, a dislocated hip and pelvis, as well as multiple fractures to one arm and leg. Organ damage included liver and other abdominal injuries and a punctured lung. He had multiple lacerations and contusions and had sustained major blood loss. His first hemoglobin reading at the hospital was 4 g/dL. Staff were made aware of the fact that he was carrying a signed medical directive requesting no blood transfusion. The request was followed. Initial treatment focused on stopping the bleeding and stabilizing major injuries. In intensive care, he was given large doses of erythropoietin and intravenous iron to build up his blood. Other treatments were used to manage his anemia. Nine days after his accident his hemoglobin had risen to 6.8 g/dL and, within another 13 days, it was back up to 11.3 g/dL. Since the time of his accident he has had 11 operations and, at time of writing, more will be required – all without the administration of any allogeneic blood.

The Impact of AIDS

The medical profession has always recognized there are problems associated with blood. Until recently, doctors generally considered these problems predominantly minor. They tended to be regarded as annoying, temporary reactions; certainly not life-threatening. Almost immediately after an operation with blood transfusion, a patient might develop a fever, or suffer some kind of allergic reaction which would pass in a moderately short time. What was not accounted for were the complications that could — and often did — manifest themselves further down the track. When those complications, like hepatitis, eventually emerged, the medical profession at large saw no connection with the earlier blood transfusion.

Even when hepatitis became recognized as a serious life-threatening transfusion complication, it failed to set off alarm bells because the disease was not perceived as a certain death sentence.

In the early 1980s this outlook changed forever. HIV/AIDS arrived and was found in the blood supply. Suddenly, here was a disease that was transmitted by blood, was incurable and, at the time, believed to be always fatal. Among its many victims were high-profile people, film stars, athletes and writers whose inevitable and untimely deaths made the front pages of newspapers around the world.

The onset of the AIDS epidemic brought great pressure upon the medical profession to modify its approach to blood transfusion. From that has emerged, for the first time, a very careful, more scientific examination of transfusion practice.

Close scrutiny of the blood supply soon showed that AIDS was not the only concern. There are many other viral, bacterial and parasitic infections that pose risks to patients. New and as yet unidentified viruses and diseases that will enter the blood supply are perhaps of even greater concern. As Dr H.R.Roberts commented in the *New England Journal of Medicine* in 1989: "No one could have predicted the tragedy of AIDS in 1978, and who can say that still unidentified but even more dangerous viruses will not contaminate the pools of plasma that are the raw materials of blood products?"

In addition to allergic and immunological reactions that have been recognized for a long time, there is now knowledge of both the short-term and long-term adverse effects of transfused blood on the immune system. Further work has been done on the changes that take place in blood when stored and the harm to patients when transfused. As the scientific examination of blood transfusion and transfusion alternatives proceeds, more and more revealing information is coming to light. We will examine some of these aspects in more detail in later chapters.

The aim of this book is to highlight the significance of the changes taking place so rapidly, and to explain how they may affect the ordinary person. In the following chapters we will examine the available options offered by bloodless surgery and provide information on how best to access them. In so doing, it is important to assess the background and reasons that have made and, pointedly, are still making such change necessary.

Historically, the human condition is one of action and reaction. Great tragedies often prompt fundamental reform. In such a context, we are all on the brink of experiencing a momentous shift in medical practice that, without question, will have enormous impact on our society and on generations to come.

Change frequently follows demand, and so it is now with the patient taking a leading role. After all, your health is really in your hands. That is as it should be – it is your body, and so your choice!

[1]   The volume in a unit of blood varies according to the component it contains and its preparation. A unit of whole blood contains the complete collection of a single donation or 'unit' of about 450 ml of blood and about 63 ml of an anticoagulant. So it is approximately half a liter or about a pint. More commonly, red blood cells (RBCs) are transfused. A unit of RBCs (composed of a single donation from which a portion of the plasma has been removed) has an additive solution and ends up with a total volume per unit ranging from some 250 to 350 ml. While other components such as platelet concentrates, plasma and clotting factors are transfused, the term 'blood transfusion' is most often used loosely to refer to the transfusion of red blood cells.

[2]   Allogeneic is a term used to describe blood, organs and tissue from another person. For many years the word 'homologous' was used, but allogeneic is now the preferred and more accurate one. It identifies the blood is from the same species but it is genetically different and individual. The authors decided to use this current word in the text to distinguish between different types of transfusion, eg., autologous (one's own) blood and non-blood volume expanders often transfused in bloodless surgery.

[3]   Some prefer the term 'transfusion-free medicine and surgery.' The authors have chosen to use the historical term that has been used in medical literature for more than 40 years and, once understood, is readily recognized.

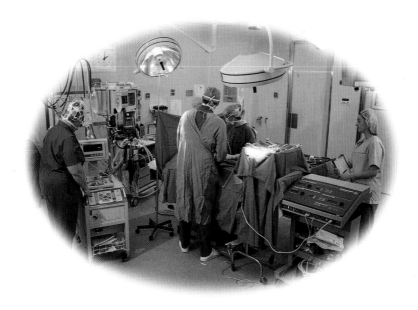

CHAPTER 2

BLOOD, THE RIVER OF LIFE

Chapter

Our 100,000-mile Lifeline

*Y*ou stay alive and well, day after day, year after year, thanks to a unique system of body components which add up to an extraordinary human performance. It's like an orchestra playing in harmony. Everything must function in concert according to carefully prescribed rules. These maintain the proper balance and rhythm essential for normal health.

Blood has been called "the river of life" for good reason. We can live without limbs and even some of our organs. But without blood, there is no human or animal life. It is the essential ingredient and driving force in a complex and integrated system which performs many vital tasks in keeping us alive and in good health.

At first glance, there is nothing obviously outstanding about the reddish liquid that flows through our veins and arteries, oxygenating and nourishing the body as it goes, rather like sap in a tree. A closer look, however, reveals an absolutely remarkable scenario.

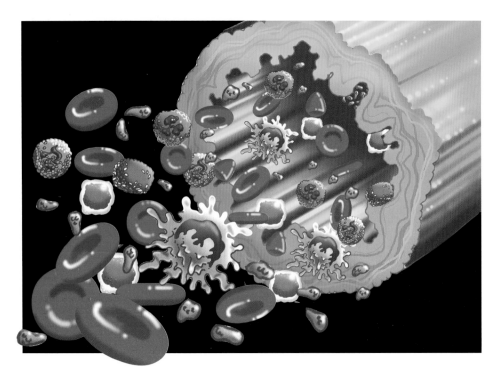

Adults have an average five to six liters of blood. It's not a lot when you think about it. Less than a bucket of water! Still, it is how these few liters are dispersed within our system that presents an amazing feat of engineering. The human heart pumps, on average, at a rate of 70 to 75 beats every minute. This is the time it takes for the blood to circulate the body, shifting five liters each time. On a normal day, some 10 tonnes of blood are moved, the equivalent of 120 tankfuls of fuel in the average six-cylinder family automobile. You don't need to be an Einstein to appreciate how much greater is the volume shifted when you exercise or run hard and your blood circulates the body every 10 seconds, or six times faster than normal!

Even more remarkable, perhaps, is the massive network of tubing through which the blood must pass on its non-stop return journey from the heart. Altogether, the combined length of the arteries, arterioles, capillaries, venules and veins within your body add up to an astonishing 100,000 miles (160,000 kilometers). Put another way, were you able to place them end to end, the distance covered would be from the Earth almost halfway to the Moon, or four times around the Earth.

The statistical extravaganza doesn't end there. In its average daily 1,440 trips around the body, blood services an estimated 75 trillion cells. To stay alive, those cells need oxygen, nutrients and fluid, all at the correct temperature and in the right pH and chemical environment. Oxygen is used by the body to "burn up" nutrients to produce the energy that sustains the life processes. From all these chemical reactions, or metabolism, there are wastes or by-products, one being carbon dioxide. For the health of the cells these need to be removed. Blood plays a key role in maintaining this constant internal environment known as *homeostasis*.

Far more than the staggering pumping paraphernalia of heart, muscles, valves, pressures and vascular activity is required, however, if the blood is to maintain its vital activity. All must be monitored via a complex circuit of sensory receptors throughout the body ensuring equilibrium and efficiency with everything working properly. A communications network, comprising the nervous and hormonal or endocrine systems, is essential for transmitting messages back to the control center. A defence shield must provide protection from invasion by disease-carrying organisms and, with 100,000 miles of plumbing, there must be in place an intricate repair mechanism to fix any ruptures. The requirements don't end there. Blood also needs one means of collecting and transporting oxygen and another that likewise collects and delivers various nutrients to the cells. Then wastes, gathered by the blood from the cells, require a purification process for expulsion via the lungs, kidneys, skin, gastro-intestinal tract and liver.

This labyrinthine method of collection, transport and delivery, begins when the blood is pumped from the right side of the heart to the lungs. There it unloads carbon dioxide collected from its previous trip around the body and loads up with a fresh supply of oxygen. Then it's back to the left side of the heart where it is pumped out via the main artery (aorta) to service all parts of the body. Arteries branch and divide into medium sized arteries. These in turn become smaller arteries, and still smaller arteries called arterioles. As the arterioles enter body tissue, they branch out again into countless microscopic vessels called capillaries. From this point the "action" begins. While the blood itself stays within the vessels, its cargo — oxygen and other substances — is squeezed by various pressures through the thin walls of the capillaries into the fluid surrounding the cells outside (interstitial or tissue fluid), and then into the cells themselves. The return journey to the heart is just as remarkable. Before leaving the tissue, groups of capillaries reunite into small veins (venules) which, in turn, merge to form progressively the larger vessels we know as veins.

Blood circulation amounts to a two-way operation. Goods for delivery — oxygen and nutrients – go out to the body's tissue mass via the capillaries, in exchange for the wastes and carbon dioxide. These, in turn are returned via the veins for dumping before the blood is re-oxygenated for the next round trip. It is an extraordinary performance which happens at least every minute of our lives!

Sadly, such a complex and efficient transport system which nourishes every cell in the body can, in some circumstances, also react against us and become an efficient carrier of disease, as we will discuss in a later chapter.

For the immediate purpose of explaining the functioning of the blood system, we will assume that the body is in normal good health. Also, for the reader to understand better why bloodless surgery is gaining pace and recognition worldwide, it is helpful to know some details about the composition of blood and the many duties its various components perform to keep the body in good health.

Blood and its Components

Blood is a complex organ made up of three distinctly different cellular components and plasma, a straw-colored fluid in which those elements and other products are suspended. The three components are red blood cells (*erythrocytes*), white blood cells (*leukocytes*) and platelets (*thrombocytes*), each with one or more specific and vital jobs to perform.

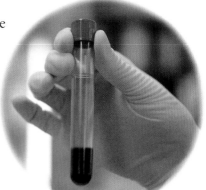

The red cells comprise 45% of total blood volume, while the white cells represent only a tiny 0.1% of volume and the platelets 0.17%. This leaves plasma with approximately 55%, providing the fluid in which the other elements are suspended to be carried around the system. Plasma, consisting largely of water (92%) also contains certain proteins with a special role to play in maintaining good health. In a pinprick of blood there are some six million red blood cells, each carrying an estimated 640 million molecules of hemoglobin. In the same amount of blood there are between 150,000 and 400,000 platelets and from 4,000 to 10,000 white blood cells.

Let us now look at the composition of blood, starting with the **red blood cells**. These are, in a sense, the star performers of the team, despite the inter-dependent nature of the overall system. Their essential role is to transport oxygen from the lungs to the body's cells (a small amount of oxygen is also dissolved in the plasma), and return to the lungs with carbon dioxide where this is expelled before the cycle begins again. Your blood contains multi-trillions of red cells, so tiny that a stack of 500 would be about one millimeter high! By strange contrast, were it possible to place each of your red blood cells on top of each other, the resultant stack would be 50,000 kilometers high. An extraordinary dimension when you consider the available five liters of source material! The red cells have a lifespan of about 120 days, which means the body has to reproduce in the bone marrow two million cells every second to replace those being retired. When needed, for example in blood loss, this red blood cell production (*erythropoiesis*) can be increased enormously – up to 10 times the usual rate.

The Makeup of Blood

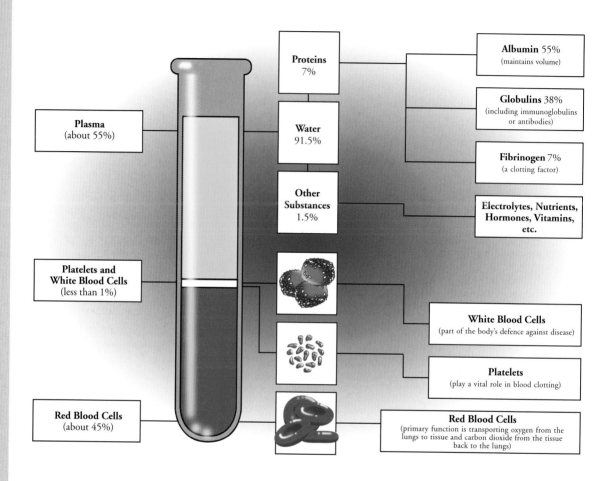

A single red blood cell is a bi-concave disc with a flexible membrane shaped rather like a doughnut with the hole filled in, or a tennis ball squashed between finger and thumb. This shape provides a larger surface-to-volume ratio than a sphere (60-70% greater), maximizing the cell's ability for gas exchange. The red cells' flexible membrane means they can change shape. This is important when it comes to their maneuvering through the microcirculation. The diameter of red blood cells is about 8 microns, whereas the minimum diameter of the capillaries through which they need to travel is about 3.5 microns. So, red blood cells need to bend and fold to squeeze through in single file, like narrow links in an endless chain.

The way the red cells collect, carry and release oxygen is equally impressive. The actual molecule within the red cell responsible for this is hemoglobin, which consists of a protein called *globin* and a pigment called *heme*, the latter containing iron.

One red blood cell carries an estimated 640 million molecules of hemoglobin and, as the cells move through the lungs, each of four iron atoms in the hemoglobin molecule "grabs", or combines with a molecule of oxygen. The significance of this is the provision of a four-fold reserve of oxygen for release into the system in the event of blood loss. In normal circumstances, the hemoglobin molecule releases only one of the four oxygen molecules it absorbs into the body tissue. However, because of the additional back-up supply, the hemoglobin molecule is able to release more oxygen to compensate when there is greater demand. We'll look at this process again shortly.

The amount of hemoglobin in an adult has for long been expressed as a measurement of grams per deciliter (g/dL) but, more recently, as grams per liter (g/L). In order not to confuse the reader, the authors have retained the more commonly used earlier g/dL measure. The average male hemoglobin level is between 14g/dL (140g/L) and 18g/dL (180g/L). For a woman it ranges from 12g/dL (120g/L) to 16 g/dL (160g/L).[1]

The **white blood cells** (produced mainly in the bone marrow) have an entirely different function from their red counterparts. Fewer in number, rounder in shape and generally larger, the white cells make up the body's first line of defence against disease and infection. Altogether there are between one and two trillion of these cells, a million of which may form every second in the bone marrow.

While numerically inferior to their red brothers, the white cells function as an amazingly complex but efficient defence force. They are rather like an army of different specialist divisions, trained and equipped to tackle every form of assault by the most devious of enemies, whether these be one or more kinds of parasite, virus, bacteria or any other disease-carrying invader. Thus different white cells have different roles. They act variously as signallers, front-line defenders, support troops and back-up heavy artillery, all with the ultimate objective of destroying the enemy. Such is the white cells' amazing versatility in recognizing, then dealing with any alien invader entering the bloodstream, that the body's immune system is often likened to the complexity and performance of the brain.

Both the **platelets** and the **plasma** play a supportive, defensive role in stopping bleeding. Platelets are tiny, short-lived (about nine days) oval-shaped discs deriving their name from their plate-like shape. They play a vital role in the proceedings that make the blood clot. When a blood vessel is cut or damaged, it immediately constricts, reducing the blood flow and blood loss.

The vessel lining is like non-stick teflon. When it is breached, platelets come in contact with substances in the ruptured vessel wall. These activate the platelets. They then change shape, enlarge and become sticky and attach themselves to the vessel's ruptured area and to each other to form an initial plug.

A process is then set off which is known as a *coagulation cascade* — a chain reaction of various chemicals in the plasma or *coagulation factors* — to form a network of fibers binding the plug into a strong clot. One substance activates another until the plasma protein, fibrinogen, is converted to an insoluble, thread-like substance called fibrin. This forms strands which fuse together the whole clot and progressively strengthen and stabilise it into a strong plug to seal the hole. When the repair work has been completed successfully, the system seems to go in reverse, breaking down the clot and dissolving it *(fibrinolysis)*. Without this remarkable mechanism, our bodies would be in danger of either bleeding to death in the first instance, or simply clogging up with an unstoppable coagulation process backing up through the system after the bleeding had long ended. This is an important area of bloodless surgery because, as you will discover later, a range of medications and techniques can stimulate and work with the coagulation system to reduce bleeding and blood loss.

Fibrinogen is just one of the three major proteins carried in plasma. (These three proteins constitute about 7% of the plasma.) Another very important protein is **albumin**. Along with electrolytes in the plasma, albumin regulates blood volume. By osmotic pressure it maintains the balance between fluid inside the blood vessels and that in the tissues surrounding the cells outside the blood vessels.

Fluid volume and pressures throughout need to be perfectly balanced to enable the heart and vascular system to pump effectively and to allow substances to move in and out of the blood vessels. For example, in acute blood loss, the rapid loss of fluid volume and blood pressure can lead to the arteries collapsing, thereby shutting off the supply of oxygen to the vital organs. This is circulatory shock.

Additionally, where there is severe blood loss and albumin levels are significantly reduced, fluid can leak from the blood vessels into the tissue fluid. This excessive accumulation of fluid in the tissue is referred to as *edema*. Pulmonary edema, or fluid on the lungs, can further compromise oxygen collection and delivery.

All these factors have special significance in bloodless surgery techniques whereby it is possible to maintain blood volume and fluid balance by transfusing appropriate non-blood fluids known as *volume expanders*.

The third major class of plasma proteins are the **globulins**, or *antibodies*, which form part of the body's defence system. In addition to food substances from digestion, including amino acids, glucose and fatty acids, plasma contains inorganic salts called *electrolytes*, that help maintain osmotic pressure and the body's acid balance. Plasma also carries hormones to control and regulate the various functions of the body and enzymes to hasten chemical reactions.

Blood Cell Development

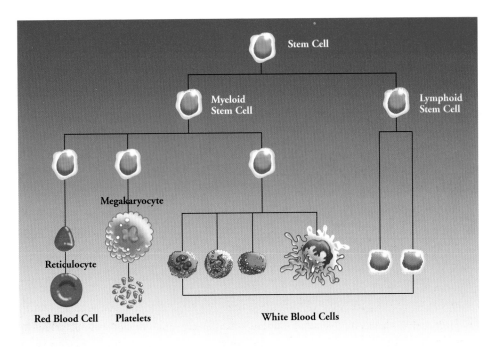

The development lines of blood cells. The intermediate forms have been left out for simplicity.

All cells have a common origin in the human marrow as a stem cell, an immature blood-forming cell. Hormones such as erythropoietin and interleukin and other stimulating factors act on the stem cells causing them to divide, multiply and mature through various stages into the different types of blood cells. Through this process they subsequently become committed to three main cell lines.

Red blood cells: Stem cells, which are stimulated by erythropoietin, develop through approximately five stages or forms to become an immature red blood cell known as a reticulocyte. The reticulocyte spends about 1-2 days in the bone marrow before being released into the bloodstream where it takes a further 1-2 days to develop into a mature red blood cell. If anemic, the body can shorten the maturation time and release reticulocytes earlier from the bone marrow. Doctors measure the percentage of reticulocytes in the bloodstream as a test of red blood cell production.

Platelets: Platelets begin with thrombopoietin driving the division and development of stem cells through about five stages into a very large cell called a megakaryocyte. This large cell then sheds fragments that form into platelets. Each megakaryocyte can produce some 4,000 platelets.

White blood cells: The third main cell line produces the various white blood cells – which include lymphocytes, monocytes and neutrophils. These form the body's immune system.

On average, 200,000 million red blood cells, 10,000 million white blood cells and 400,000 million platelets are formed daily by this process. When the need arises, the body can increase the production of one or more cell lines 10-fold or more.

Blood: Mystique and Mistakes

Understanding what you know now about blood took the human race centuries to learn. It wasn't until the early 1900s that blood types and groups were discovered. A lot more has come to light about blood in the past 50 years.

Not surprisingly, humans have always viewed blood with awe and mysticism. Hence when a means was developed to transfuse blood from one human to another, it was seen as *the gift of life*. History is full of examples of the diverse ways in which blood was viewed, used and abused. Its perceived qualities have varied from being a source of physical strength to even the more mystical. Roman gladiators would drink their vanquished opponents' blood to give them extra vigor. Other cultures, such as Africans and American Indians, mingled their blood in rituals to become blood brothers. Blood has been used as nourishment and bonding agents. It has been used to seal treaties. It has also been used to poison.

The supposed healing powers of blood give it an equally varied and long history of use in medicine. A physician of the 7th century BC used blood to treat the son of Assyrian King Esarhaddon. He reported to the king: "Shamash-shumu-ukin is doing much better; the king, my lord, can be happy. Starting with the 22nd day I give (him) blood to drink, he will drink (it) for three days. For three more days I shall give (him blood) for internal application."

Numerous early reports tell how blood was used to treat epilepsy. A second-century physician, Aretaeus of Cappadocia, described the treatment thus: "I have seen persons holding a cup below the wound of a man recently slaughtered, and drinking a draught of the blood!" Similarly, Tertullian, of the third century, reported how epileptics drank the fresh blood of slain gladiators.

Blood was also used in 1483 to treat the dying Louis XI of France. Historian Reay Tannahill wrote: "Every day he grew worse, and the medicines profited him nothing, though of a strange character; for he vehemently hoped to recover by the human blood which he took and swallowed from certain children."

For almost 2,500 years medicine took blood from patients by a practice called *bleeding* or *bloodletting*. It was believed disease was caused by an imbalance of fluids, or *humors*. Bloodletting, it was thought, would remove the "bad humors". Consequently, doctors bled patients to treat a broad spectrum of complaints including headaches, plague, broken bones and, sometimes, even to stop bleeding.

Opinions vary on when the very first blood transfusion was performed. Some suggest the Ancient Egyptians were the first to practice it; others believe it was the Incas of South America. Yet again, others credit Pope Innocent VII with being the first patient in 1492. A contemporary account reads: "Meanwhile, in the city [of Rome] tribulations and deaths have never ceased; for, first of all, three ten-year-old boys, from whose veins a certain Jewish physician (who had promised that the pope would be restored to health) extracted blood, died without delay. For, in fact, the Jew had told them he wanted to heal the pontiff, if only he could have a certain quantity of human blood and indeed young; which, therefore, he ordered to be extracted from three boys, to whom after the blood-letting he gave a ducat for each; and shortly thereafter they died. The Jew indeed fled, and the pope was not healed."

In point of fact, the pontiff may not have been transfused intravenously, because the technology enabling direct injection into the veins had yet to be developed. In 1628, English physician William Harvey first mapped the blood circulatory system. Twenty-eight years later, the eminent British scientist and mathematician, Christopher Wren, developed a means of injecting directly into the blood vessels. He used a sharpened goose quill attached to an animal bladder. In early experiments physicians injected a variety of substances into their patients such as milk, dye, wine and opium. These practices eventually led to transfusing blood, firstly animal blood into other animals, then animal blood into humans.

Transfusion with Animal Blood

In 1665, Oxford scientist John Wilkins and English doctor Richard Lower began experiments in transfusing blood from one dog to another. Others followed. In France, physician Jean Baptiste Denys began experiments in this field and transfused calves' blood into dogs.

The first documented transfusion of animal blood into humans was by Denys in 1667, when he treated a 16-year-old youth tormented with a violent fever. He first removed three ounces of blood from the boy, then transfused him with nine ounces (a cupful) of lamb's blood. In the same year Richard Lower

32

transfused lamb's blood into a former minister described as being "crack'd a little in the head."

Interestingly, the early blood transfusions were used not to treat blood loss, but psychiatric and emotional problems. The popular belief was that personality, characteristics and temperament were carried in the blood.

Denys continued human transfusions, his most famous being in 1667-68 when he transfused calves' blood into a 34-year-old man to treat his insanity. The patient, a Parisian named Antoine Mauroy, suffered frenzies during which he would batter his wife, strip off his clothes and run naked through the streets, setting fire to houses on the way. The doctor hoped that calves' blood "by its mildness and freshness might possibly allay the heat and ebullition of the patient's blood."

Denys believed animal blood was purer than the human variety because of man's "debauchery and irregularities in eating and drinking." If a man could successfully imbibe milk from an animal as a nutrient, he reasoned, why not animal blood intravenously?

Denys transfused Mauroy twice, initially, after which his patient complained about a feeling of heat and pain travelling up his arm. The man's pulse began to race. He started to sweat profusely; complained of severe back pain and was nauseous. He vomited, had a severe nose-bleed and then experienced breathing difficulties. Denys stopped the transfusion. The next day Mauroy "made a great glass of urine with a color as black as if it had been mixed with the soot of a chimney."

The experimenting physician was not to know it, but his patient was undergoing an episode of near-fatal hemolytic transfusion reaction, caused when a person receives incompatible blood. The body reacts by producing antibodies to destroy the invading foreign cells. In the ensuing battle, millions of red cells are destroyed, with the debris and toxins ending up in the kidneys where they trigger inflammation and pain. The oxidized hemoglobin turns the urine black.

Mauroy managed to survive, but in three months his condition had deteriorated again and Denys was asked to carry out a third transfusion. This time when the doctor tried to transfuse him, the patient convulsed and went into shock, dying the following day. The man's death resulted in a charge of murder being brought against Denys, from which he was later exonerated. It happened that Mauroy's wife was poisoning the patient and it was she who ultimately ended up in the dock.

As a consequence of this and other tragic instances, the Faculty of Medicine in Paris pronounced that transfusion was dangerous and scientifically unsound. In 1670, the French parliament banned the practice. After two more deaths from animal blood transfusions in Rome, the Pope ordered the procedure stopped in most parts of Europe. Meanwhile, England also quietly discontinued these experiments, with the Royal Society in London ultimately outlawing the practice.

First Human Blood Transfusion

The therapy of transfusing blood remained dormant until the early 1800s, when the medical profession gained an increased understanding of physiology, the role of blood and the dangers of hemorrhage. English obstetrician James Blundell recognized the dangers of hemorrhage following childbirth and introduced blood transfusion as a means of replacing lost blood. He believed only human blood should be transfused into humans and performed the first human blood transfusion in 1818, from which the patient died. Ten years later, however, Blundell carried out the first successful human blood transfusion. He went on to become noted for developing means of returning the patient's own blood following hemorrhage at childbirth. This earned him the title of "father of modern autotransfusion" (transfusing a patient's own blood).

Transfusions were used only sporadically during the 19th century, becoming more popular in the latter half. At this time doctors knew nothing about storing blood, so it was necessary to transfuse direct from donor to recipient, with one person's vessels either stitched to the other's, or the blood transported through a glass tube or injected by syringe. With doctors bereft of knowledge about preventing blood clotting, problems of clotting in the apparatus were common. Additionally, physicians had no understanding of different blood types. Consequently, the majority of people died from the experience. It wasn't until the 20th century that blood transfusion began to gain wide acceptance.

Modern History

A breakthrough in scientific knowledge about blood came in 1901 through the work of Austrian pathologist Karl Landsteiner. Then a research assistant at the Vienna Pathological Institute, Landsteiner discovered blood varied from person to person and would react when combined. Initially, he identified three major types: A, B and O. Later he found others. Most important of all, he discovered that if blood from one group was transfused into a person with a different blood group, the recipient's blood would mount an immune response of antibodies and attack the introduced cells. Landsteiner was appointed Professor of Pathology at the University of Vienna in 1909 and, in 1930, was awarded the Nobel Prize for his discovery of the major blood groups.

It had taken almost 20 years for Landsteiner's initial discovery to be accepted and for blood typing to become common practice in blood transfusion. In the meantime, many patients continued to have serious transfusion reactions. Death was commonplace. In 1915, American doctor Richard Lewishon achieved wide recognition when he developed a means of stopping blood from clotting. The secret was the anticoagulant, sodium citrate. Initially, this was used simply to prevent blood from clotting in the apparatus of direct donor-to-patient transfusions. It was this discovery that later made it possible to store blood in bottles without it clotting, which, in turn, allowed it to be transported.

Then came the bloodbath of World War I. Doctors began to experience and analyze first-hand the connection, made 100 years earlier by Blundell, between blood volume loss and death. Soldiers who lost a significant amount of blood from injuries were dying from lack of fluid volume rather than a compromised oxygen supply due to reduced red blood cells. When blood volume fell to the point where the blood pressure dropped, their vascular system collapsed and their heart and circulatory system were unable to function. The soldiers were dying essentially from circulatory shock. What they needed was fluid to restore their blood volume and blood pressure, not red blood cells.

Doctors experimented with transfusing a number of fluids as volume expanders, including saline, a water and salt solution. However, these were only partially effective because the fluids they were using didn't stay in the system long enough and many believed that whole blood was still needed.

It was the Russians who, in the 1930s, realized they could store blood and transport it to their patients. They would drain blood from cadavers, store it, then transport it country-wide to be transfused. Experiments were also said to have been done with cadaver blood in the USA, Canada and India. Despite some deaths and reactions, it was considered a "safe" and "lifesaving" procedure and opened the way for blood storage on a large scale. This led to the establishment in Moscow of the world's first institute dedicated to the study of blood. Ironically, one of its founders later died from a transfusion reaction.

American doctor Bernard Fantus (pictured right) is credited with establishing the first "blood bank" in the US in 1937. Blood collected from donors had sodium citrate added before being stored in refrigerators.

Two years later, World War II erupted and blood once again flowed on battlefields. Blood was now collected, stored and mobilized on a massive scale, with an estimated 13 million units subsequently transfused. During this period medical science developed the ability to separate blood into its individual components. Plasma

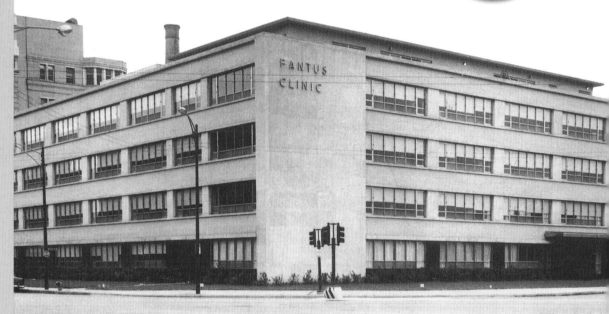

The Chicago Fantus Clinic – the first so-called "blood bank" in the US – 1937

was withdrawn and used as a volume expander. Further scientific research enabled the separating of proteins from plasma, a process known as fractionation. The albumin collected by this process was also used as a volume expander.

After the war ended in 1945, surgeons who had become accustomed to using banked blood promoted the establishment of civilian blood banks. These, coupled with the identification of blood types, anti-coagulants and preservatives, encouraged a general acceptance that blood was a "safe" and relatively risk-free therapy. As a consequence, blood transfusion became common practice in surgery and medical treatment, allowing larger and more complex operations to be performed. Indeed, blood transfusion emerged as "standard practice," its use spreading beyond more complex surgical operations to all procedures. Blood became ordered as a standby provision. So common was its use, blood was often given as a "top-up," allegedly to make the patient feel better.

The Future of Transfusion

For 2,500 years, medicine employed bloodletting. It was practiced by Egyptians, Greeks, Romans and, in Western medicine, right through to the 20th century. It became standard practice and was held in high regard, as evidenced by the name chosen for the prestigious British medical journal, *The Lancet*. More than that, it was viewed as a miraculous cure. In 1642, Dr Guy Patin, Dean of the Faculty of Medicine in Paris, wrote: "There is no remedy in the world which works as many miracles as bleeding". And yet even though it was to become one of the longest lasting medical practices, there was never any evidence that bleeding actually worked or did any good.

The 20th century in a sense saw the procedure reversed with blood transfusion becoming standard practice. Basically, the emphasis changed from taking blood out to putting it in. Like bloodletting before it, transfusion was also described as a "miraculous cure." Even today, the efficacy of blood transfusion has yet to be proved scientifically. Many blood transfusions have been, and continue to be, administered based on traditional practice rather than scientific evidence.

History shows that change comes with challenge; action prompting reaction. New solutions have to be found to prevent disasters recurring. It has certainly been thus in the medical world where events have sparked research, discovery and ultimately change. Bloodless surgery is a dramatic case in point. Here medicine is reacting to one of the most serious health threats of modern times. Today's concerns had their first public impact in the 1980s with the dawning of AIDS, forcing a more critical look at blood transfusion and the need for alternatives.

In assessing the long and varied history of blood and its many applications – whether misplaced, mythological or medical – the question now posed is: How much longer will it be before transfusion becomes yet another closed chapter in the still unfolding story?

[1] Another common measurement of the hemoglobin level is referred to as the hematocrit, sometimes 'crit' for short. Hematocrit measures the percentage of red blood cells in the blood. Normally the red blood cells make up about 45% of the blood volume and so a normal hematocrit is about 45%. Again this varies between men and women. A male's normal hematocrit is between 40 - 54% and a female's between 38 - 47%. By multiplying the hemoglobin value by three, one can do a quick, rough conversion to hematocrit. Conversely, if you divide the hematocrit by three you are able to convert it to a hemoglobin value. If your doctor tells you your hematocrit is 30%, a quick calculation will tell you that your hemoglobin is about 10 g/dL.

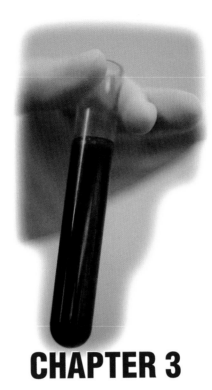

CHAPTER 3

WHEN BLOOD IS A KILLER

Chapter

River of Life; Carrier of Disease

We have explained blood's unique characteristics and life-sustaining function as a carrier of sustenance to every cell in the body. Now we need to examine its less appealing characteristics. Blood is also the carrier of disease which can be debilitating and sometimes life-threatening. Of equal concern are other negative effects of transfused blood, such as slower recovery after an operation and, more serious still, a compromised immune system.

It is recognized there have always been problems associated with blood. The disease we now know as hepatitis, caused by an infectious virus, has been the scourge of armies and populations for centuries, going back to Babylonian times. For decades it was simply known as jaundice. The disease – with early symptoms of yellowing complexion followed by liver failure – often resulted from lack of hygiene. In the worst possible conditions, such as on battlefields, it rampaged through the ranks of frontline soldiers. Jaundice decimated Napoleon's army during its Egyptian campaign. It created problems during the American Civil War and, indeed, in all the major conflicts of the 19th and 20th centuries. At best, it left its victims very sick; at worst, it killed them.

Recognition of blood as a carrier of disease took on an extra dimension with the development of blood transfusion. At the time of the early attempts at transfusion, doctors were preoccupied with solving the complications associated with adverse reactions, such as those described in the previous chapter. They had little understanding of disease, its causes and transmission. It wasn't until the late 1800s and the early 1900s that the role of bacteria and viruses in disease transmission was discovered. In 1915, syphilis was the first bacterium to be identified as being transmissible by blood. Malaria, caused by a parasite, was another blood-transmitted disease recognized around this time.

In 1885, hepatitis became the first virus confirmed as blood-borne. However, it was not until 1943 that an American, Dr Paul Beeson, linked the transmission of hepatitis with blood transfusion. In *The Journal of the American Medical Association*, he reported patients were coming down with the disease one to four months after transfusion. The long incubation period of this virus had hidden its danger in transfusion for decades. In time, it was quite apparent there were different types of hepatitis, and these became officially designated by the letters of the alphabet.

During World War II and, subsequently, the Korean War in the early 1950s, thousands of soldiers contracted hepatitis from transfusion. In the 1970s, hepatitis B became a serious transfusion complication described by some as an "epidemic." In 1975, various authorities estimated post-transfusion hepatitis B cases in the United States had reached 17,000 a year, with as many as 3,500 or more deaths. Some suggested the figure could have been ten times that number. This, despite a blood-screening test, first developed in 1972 and then improved three years later. With further testing and screening vigilance, the number of hepatitis B cases decreased. Then another deadly form of the virus was detected. Initially labelled "non-A non-B" hepatitis, it eventually became identified as hepatitis C. This was to be the new wave of the disease that would eventually progress into a world community health problem. A report published in 1998 estimated four million people in the US were suffering from hepatitis C, with 8,000 – 10,000 deaths a year from long-term infection. Among its victims were the poor and the prominent alike. The world was shocked when the international star, Danny Kaye, died. He had contracted hepatitis C from a blood transfusion received four years earlier.

AIDS, the Killer

Despite the number of people who contracted hepatitis from blood transfusions, the disease did not have the public impact AIDS had when it arrived in the early 1980s. Initially, many felt it was confined to certain sub-cultures, in particular homosexual men. AIDS, the acronym for acquired immune deficiency syndrome, was a disease that appeared to be universally fatal. In 1983, it was confirmed AIDS could be transmitted by the therapeutic use of blood and blood products. Four years later the American Association of Blood Banks, the largest blood collecting organization in the US, published a book that, in part, examined the history of donor programs following World War II. The book also addressed the problems the association faced functioning in an increasingly complex scientific and social environment.

"But then the fabric of this gradually evolving tapestry was dramatically, suddenly and irreversibly rent by the appearance of acquired immune deficiency syndrome

(AIDS)," wrote contributing author Dr Donald R. Avoy, Medical Director of the Health Assurance Corporation, Sunnyvale, California. "Almost as soon as the original risk groups were defined, the unthinkable occurred: the demonstration that this potentially lethal disease could and was being transmitted by the volunteer blood supply. This was the most bitter of all medical ironies; that the precious life-giving gift of blood could turn out to be an instrument of death."

All of this had a dramatic effect on the public's perception of blood transfusion. It also forced the medical profession to reassess its transfusion practices and search for better approaches. Celebrities were getting AIDS. High-profile people were getting AIDS. From the little girl next door to the corporate leader, it was a disease that didn't differentiate between class, sex or occupation. It was a disease to which everyone could relate. And it was killing people. Whole communities in Africa and Asia were being threatened. By 1995, an estimated 20,000 Americans had contracted AIDS from blood transfusions.

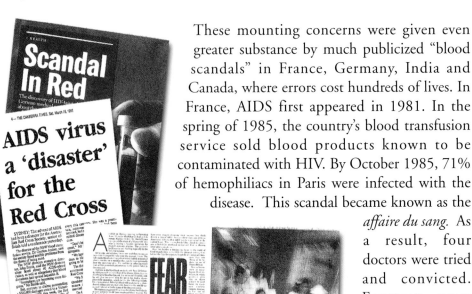

These mounting concerns were given even greater substance by much publicized "blood scandals" in France, Germany, India and Canada, where errors cost hundreds of lives. In France, AIDS first appeared in 1981. In the spring of 1985, the country's blood transfusion service sold blood products known to be contaminated with HIV. By October 1985, 71% of hemophiliacs in Paris were infected with the disease. This scandal became known as the *affaire du sang*. As a result, four doctors were tried and convicted. Fourteen years after the event, the scandal re-emerged with another court case. This time a former prime minister and two of his cabinet were charged with manslaughter. The former leader and one of his ministers were subsequently acquitted. One-time health minister, Edmund Herve, was convicted for his role in the contamination of seven people. However, in what the media described as a "compromise verdict," Herve received no penalty.

Meanwhile, in Germany in 1993, investigators found that a blood-supply company took short cuts in screening. On occasions the company had failed to screen blood for HIV. Authorities traced batches of the blood distributed to 86 hospitals. The company had also shipped blood products to Austria, Greece and Saudi Arabia. Records revealed that Portugal, Sweden, Italy, Switzerland, France, the Netherlands and Britain could have received blood products from the same source.

Indian officials ordered a Bombay blood bank closed in 1995. Their action followed charges that the bank had supplied HIV-infected blood to city hospitals between 1992 and 1994. A number of employees were also accused of selling HIV-infected blood on the black market. Shortly thereafter a Canadian judicial inquiry began examining reports that 1,200 people had been infected with HIV and up to 60,000 with hepatitis C.

AIDS is caused by one of two human viruses, HIV-1 and HIV-2, each of which breaks down the body's immune system and exposes its victims to all sorts of opportunistic diseases. Despite intense scientific research, it was not until the mid-1980s that HIV was identified. In 1985, scientists developed an effective test to detect HIV antibodies in donor blood.

This blood test, along with donor screening, has significantly reduced the chances of HIV/AIDS being transmitted by blood in many countries. Australia, for example, managed to avoid any HIV transmission through transfusion for 15 years. However, in July 1999, a stunned nation learned that a 14-year-old Melbourne schoolgirl, the daughter of a surgeon, had contracted the disease from a blood transfusion during surgery. In the United States it is reported that there are probably fewer than 20 transfusion-related cases a year. Of course, for those 20 people this improved statistic is of little comfort. Other countries have not had as much success and are still reporting cases of AIDS transmitted via screened blood.

What Screening Cannot See

"Major infectious agents still elude the most sensitive assays, while less-common infectious agents, such as parvoviruses, spirochetes, parasites, bacteria and possibly, viruses with prolonged incubation periods, cannot be eliminated by practical screening tests."

Harvey G. Klein MD
Department of Transfusion Medicine, Warren G. Magnuson Clinical Center, National Institutes of Health, Bethesda Maryland.
Allogeneic Transfusion Risks in the Surgical Patient. *The American Journal of Surgery* 1995;170(Suppl 6A):21S-26S

"Although many measures have been taken to reduce the risks of blood transfusion, and although sophisticated technology will continue to improve its safety, it is not possible to provide a blood supply with zero risk."

Practice Parameter for the Use of Red Blood Cell Transfusions. Developed by the Red Blood Cell Administration Practice Guideline Development Task Force of the College of American Pathologists.
Archives of Pathology and Laboratory Medicine 1998;122:130-138

What needs to be understood is that most screening of donor blood involves testing for antibodies, not the virus itself. This is not a foolproof means of identifying a disease in its early stages. Such tests are applied to detect HIV-1 and 2, the hepatitis C virus and human T-cell lymphotropic virus type 1 (HTLV-1). However, there is a period between when a person is exposed to the virus and when he or she develops antibodies, referred to as the "window" period. With HIV this period may be from two to six weeks and up to several months. Some reports have even indicated window periods, in rare situations, lasting several years. This means donor blood infected by HIV may show no signs of antibodies at the time of testing and thus go undetected. There have also been reports of silent infectious conditions that prevent victims from mounting a sufficiently strong antibody response to be detected.

To cover the window period, donors are asked to complete questionnaires and sign a written statement to the effect that their lifestyle within a designated period hasn't placed them at high risk of acquiring an infection which could then be passed on by transfusion. Nevertheless, the ultimate test of this depends on the donor's attitude and honesty. Further complicating this system is the possibility of concealed activity on the part of the donor's partner.

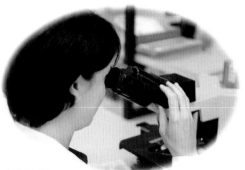

New genetic fingerprinting tests called NAT (nucleic acid testing) are undergoing experimentation. These detect viral genes and hold promise of reducing – some have suggested by about 40% – the window period by detecting viral presence in blood earlier. However, this new technology comes at much greater cost and it takes two to three days to perform the test.

Additionally, there can be human error. Even in recent times, banks have had to contact blood recipients to notify them that blood products may have been improperly tested and, consequently, they may have received contaminated blood. Such a warning was sent to people in New York and New Jersey who received blood between 1991 and 1996, in addition to which there have been regular US reports of large quantities of blood infected with viruses slipping undetected through the system every year.

Further clouding an accurate picture of the true incidence of diseases is the incubation period of some of these viruses. This should not be confused with the "window" period. The incubation period refers to the time between being exposed to the virus and the disease manifesting itself with symptoms. For example, the incubation period for AIDS is variable, with a reported seven-year average in adults.

As already described, while the development of screens has dramatically reduced the transmission of disease by blood, screens have not completely eliminated the risk. They are not foolproof. Blood banks make it very clear in their literature to potential recipients that while donor blood has never been safer, it cannot be guaranteed 100% safe. One service warns: "The risk of transmitting infectious agents is present. Careful donor selection and available laboratory tests do not completely eliminate the hazard." Patients are advised "inappropriate transfusions should be avoided and autologous (one's own predonated blood) transfusions should be considered when feasible."

The present estimated risk of contracting AIDS through blood varies dramatically from country to country, running anywhere between 1 in 200,000 units transfused to 1 in 2 million. On the other hand, the risk of contracting hepatitis B this way is greater with estimates between 1 in 30,000 to 1 in 250,000, while the hepatitis C risk estimates range from 1 in 30,000 to 1 in 150,000. Of course, if a person receives more than one unit, then the risk equation increases. The risk is also cumulative – that is, they all add up. If one calculates the risk of HIV plus hepatitis B plus hepatitis C plus cytomegalovirus, etc., it has been estimated that the risk of contracting a serious or fatal transfusion-transmitted disease is about three in every 10,000 units. According to another estimate, the mortality rate from all known infectious risks is 29 to 103 deaths per million units (there are 11 - 12 million units of red blood cells transfused each year in the US.)

AIDS has caused widespread fear of blood. Experts argue that with all the associated media hype, AIDS has hijacked public attention to such an extent that the possibility of even greater threats in the offing is yet to be properly appreciated. The fact is, there are many other viral, bacterial and parasitic diseases transmitted by blood.

Some of the potentially transmitted viral, parasitic & bacterial diseases

- HIV
- Hepatitis
- HTLV
- Cytomegalovirus
- Epstein-Barr
- Parvovirus B19
- Prion Diseases
  (eg. Creutzfeldt-Jakob disease)
- TT-Virus
- Human Herpesvirus–8
- Borna Disease Virus
- Types, subtypes and mutant and divergent strains of the above
- The next virus

- Trypanosoma cruzi
  (Chagas' Disease)
- Malaria
- Toxoplasmosis
- Typhus
- Babesiosis
- Borrelia
- Filariasis
- Leishmaniasis
- Syphilis
- Bartonella
- Brucella
- Salmonellosis & Typhoid Fever
- Yersinia

Hepatitis Viruses and Other Diseases

Hepatitis, or inflammation of the liver, has a number of causes, the most common being viruses. Others include chemicals, drugs and alcohol. The word *hepatitis* is derived from the Greek words *hepat* (liver) and *itis* (inflammation).

The main viruses causing hepatitis are designated by letters of the alphabet. So far, hepatitis types A to G have been identified. Less common causes are from viral infections such as yellow fever and cytomegalovirus. Other viruses possibly linked with hepatitis are being investigated.

At the time of publication, hepatitis G had been identified and hepatitis H was suspected. Some authorities have suggested there may not be enough letters in the alphabet to identify what lies ahead.

The list of hepatitis viruses continues to grow:

Hepatitis A: It is rarely transmitted by blood transfusion (1 in 1 million units). Its transmission is via fecal matter of an infected person. It results from close person-to- person contact, poor hygiene, contaminated utensils, food or water. It does not lead to chronic disease. The symptoms of nausea and pain in the liver and stomach usually last for three weeks, but can persist for as long as six months.

Hepatitis B: It is primarily transmitted through contaminated blood or blood products, through sexual contact (heterosexual or homosexual) and through sharing drug needles. About 35% of persons infected develop acute disease and 1 to 10 percent develop chronic disease that can lead to cirrhosis and liver cancer.

Hepatitis C: The most life-threatening of the hepatitis viruses so far identified. It is spread primarily through direct contact with infected blood, such as through blood transfusion or exposure to contaminated needles. *Some 85% of infections become chronic, 20% lead to cirrhosis, and 1% to 5% result in hepatocellular carcinoma (liver cancer). The combined mortality from cirrhosis and hepatocellular carcinoma is 14.5% over a period ranging from 21 to 28 years.*

Hepatitis D: This develops as a co-infection with the hepatitis B virus, making those symptoms more severe. It is spread through contaminated blood and needles and, unlike hepatitis B, rarely through sexual contact.

Hepatitis E: This is similar to hepatitis A and does not lead to chronic infections. It occurs mostly in developing countries where consumption of fecal-contaminated water can cause epidemics.

Hepatitis F: Like hepatitis A, it is transmitted by fecal contamination, and does not appear to lead to chronic illness.

Hepatitis G: It is transmitted by blood and can cause both acute and chronic hepatitis. It can be transmitted simultaneously with hepatitis B and C and result in co-infection. Its long-term clinical consequences are not fully known.

With each of these viruses there are also sub-types and divergent strains. For example, scientists have for some time recognised HIV Type 1 and Type 2. But recently in Europe, it was reported that HIV Type 1 Sub-type O had been identified. There are said to be at least six different types (genotypes) of hepatitis C, with more than 30 different subtypes. All this highlights that the ever-mutating viruses make it extremely challenging for the screening process.

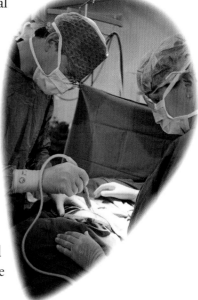

Of even greater concern than those viral, bacterial and parasitic diseases, which have been identified, are the ones that remain unknown. This raises a vital question: Could other viruses, every bit as threatening as AIDS or hepatitis, enter the blood system unidentified? This is no idle conjecture.

In 1997, scientists reported on a new virus (TT-virus) in patients with post-transfusion non-A-G hepatitis. Further research has found a high prevalence of this virus in those suffering with cirrhosis and fulminant liver failure of unknown origin, together with others who have had blood transfusion. Further work is needed to determine the TT-virus' role in causing disease.

Other viruses, such as human herpesvirus-8 (HHV-8) and borna disease virus have just emerged. In recent times a new group of poorly understood infectious agents called *prions* have attracted considerable scientific attention. These are neither virus nor bacteria, but appear to be infectious protein. At least six of these have been identified. One is known as Creutzfeldt-Jakob Disease (CJD), the human form of Mad Cow Disease. CJD attacks the brain, creating sponge-like holes which ultimately lead to dementia and death.

There is still much debate about whether or not CJD and a new strain, new variant CJD (nvCJD) can be transmitted by blood. A disturbing aspect of the disease is its long incubation period which, some have suggested, can be up to 30 years before it manifests itself. Meanwhile, equally disturbing are reports from around the world, including the United Kingdom, that thousands of patients have been given blood contaminated with CJD. Consequently, many thousands of units of blood have been recalled.

More recently, countries including the US, Canada and New Zealand have issued guidelines banning potential blood donors who have spent six or more cumulative months in Britain between January 1, 1980, and December 31, 1996. Other countries are currently considering similar action to reduce the risk of transmitting new variant CJD.

The intensification of those diseases which already pose serious health threats is another alarm point. In this category is malaria. For years, malaria has caused widespread devastation among rural populations, particularly in the developing world. Annually, three million people die from the disease worldwide. Malaria can be passed on by blood. There is, therefore, a major risk of contracting it via blood transfusions in most developing tropical countries. Reports indicate that 15% of the blood donor pool in some parts of Africa is infected.

At present, hepatitis C remains the most threatening of all the viral diseases, with the long-term potential to be even more deadly than AIDS. Today, it affects four times more people than HIV does in the United States. Worldwide, an estimated 200 million people are its victims, many of whom were given blood transfusions before blood banks began screening in the early 1990s. A 1998 University of Florida study based on projected infection rates has suggested hepatitis C infections will bring more than a five-fold increase in the demand for liver transplants during the first eight years of the new millennium. The study also predicts the number of Americans who will die from the disease in that period will treble to 30,000 a year, creating a huge extra burden on the country's health resources. In 1998, US Surgeon General David Satcher estimated health care costs for hepatitis C were already more than $600 million a year.

Some four million people in the United States have contracted the virus, with an estimated 28,000 to 180,000 new cases each year. But there could be many thousands more unaware that they have the disease, given the fact that it can lie dormant and undetected for as long as 20 years, and possibly longer. In 1998, the US government ordered a mailing campaign to notify nearly 300,000 people who might have been accidentally infected after receiving blood transfusions from donors who had since tested positive. These people received blood before June 1992 when the most reliable screening tests were initiated. At the time, former US Surgeon General, Everett C. Koop said: "We stand at the precipice of a grave threat to our public health . . . it affects people from all walks of life, in every state, in every country. And unless we do something about hepatitis C soon, it will kill more people than AIDS."

Studies have shown that hepatitis C contracted through blood transfusion (an estimated 7% of all hepatitis C cases) may be more aggressive with more severe liver damage than when contracted via other modes of transmission.

"Current screening and testing methods, while extremely effective, do not necessarily protect the blood from 'emerging agents' such as Trypanosoma Cruzi [Chagas' disease], or from mutant microbes, such as HIV type O, no longer detected by specific testing methods."

Harvey G. Klein MD
Department of Transfusion Medicine, Warren G. Magnuson Clinical Center, National Institutes of Health, Bethesda Maryland
Proceedings of a Symposium: New Insights Into the Management of Anemia in the Surgical Patient. *The American Journal of Medicine* 1996; 101(suppl 2A):12S-15S

"Finally, there is the issue of preparing for the unknown. This HIV caught plasma fractionators unawares, and so might another equally dangerous virus in the future. However, not only is it very difficult to be prepared for an unknown hazard but also there is no assurance

that the additional 'safeguards' developed would be effective."

Dr D.P. Thomas.
Viral contamination of blood products. *The Lancet*
1994;343(8913):1583-4

Special Risks for Women

The risks associated with transfused blood have particular significance for women. Hundreds of thousands of women each year face the possibility of surgery for gynecological cancer. In 1997, there were an estimated 424,800 new cases of genital tract cancer in the USA. Gynecologic cancer surgery carries the potential for significant blood loss and transfusion. Extremely high-risk procedures, including radical hysterectomy and extensive surgery for advanced cancer of the ovaries, liver, diaphragm and so on, have a blood loss varying between two and six units.

It is understandable, then, that before 1992 when more reliable screening became available for hepatitis C, women represented a large proportion of Americans who became infected with the virus after blood transfusion. Many of them received transfusions during cesarean section childbirth, often while under sedation and without their knowledge.

A 1993 study published in the American *Journal of Reproductive Medicine* indicated that only one in four women who received blood while giving birth during a cesarean section realized she had been transfused. The study estimated that 250,000 women might have contracted the hepatitis C virus in this way.

In October 1998, the executive director of a leading US women's health group urged the federal government to take a stronger lead in educating and alerting women to the potentially fatal consequences of hepatitis C. Phyllis Greenberger, president of the Society for the Advancement of Women's Health Research, described the virus as "the next major health crisis women are facing."

In a widely published statement Greenberger said: "Women have special risk factors for this disease and, because the symptoms are mostly silent, the federal government has a particular responsibility to alert women at risk."

Transfusion Reactions and Complications

The transmission of infectious diseases is the most widely held fear across the board in the community when it comes to public knowledge about transfusions. However, there is an ever-growing list of other adverse transfusion reactions, largely unappreciated by the general public. Some are mild and relatively harmless; others severe and potentially fatal. An authoritative estimate suggests that one in five of all transfusions has some adverse effect on the patient. It is also being suggested by specialists that every transfusion is associated with some sort of reaction.

The following list gives the principal hazards and side-effects of blood transfusion.

- Transmission of infectious disease
- Acute hemolytic reactions
- Febrile reactions
- Transfusion-associated acute lung injury
- Allergic reactions
- Delayed hemolytic reactions
- Alloimmunization
- Graft-versus-host disease
- Posttransfusion purpura
- Immunomodulation
  - increased postoperative infection
  - increased cancer recurrence, decreased survival
  - more rapid progression of HIV
  - activation of latent viruses
  - poorer wound healing
- Non-immune hemolysis
- Bacterial contamination
- Microaggregates
- Circulatory overload
- Coagulopathy
- Iron overload

- Metabolic complications:
  - Hypothermia
  - Citrate toxicity
  - Acidosis
- Compromise of oxygen transport
  - Biophysical & biochemical changes
- Depression of erythropoiesis
- Multi-organ failure

Immune Suppression

Just when concerns about HIV and hepatitis C transmission began to fade because of improved testing, another issue arose: **immune suppression from transfusion**. Researchers have discovered that blood transfusion suppresses many facets of the body's immune function (referred to as transfusion-associated immunomodulation, or TRIM). Some of these effects are short-term, others long-term, and some even permanent. The experts have suggested TRIM makes the body more vulnerable to postoperative infection and increased cancer recurrence. Clearly, this is no minor issue.

Dr Paul Tartter, of the Mount Sinai Medical Center, New York, made an incisive observation back in 1992 when he described blood transfusion as the "earliest form of transplantation." Writing in the *Journal of Intensive Care Medicine*, Tartter referred to the suppression of many facets of the immune function that followed transfusion. Some functions, he noted, returned to normal in "hours or weeks." He emphasized, however, that there was evidence of permanent alteration to immune function. Immune inhibition 18 months after transfusion had been noted in patients undergoing surgery for inflammatory bowel disease. He added: "Lymphocyte (immune cells) inhibition has also been observed up to 30 years after transfusion in women who received blood for Rh incompatibility as neonates (newborns)."

Infection is unquestionably a major cause of complications and death following surgery. Because of this, immune suppression from blood transfusion may well be the most serious life-threatening outcome of the therapy. Evidence suggests immune suppression complications slow the healing process and result in the use of significantly more antibiotics. As stated earlier, a patient who has undergone allogeneic blood transfusion is generally more likely to spend longer in hospital than the person who has not.

In a compelling article in the journal, *Seminars in Hematology*, Professor Neil Blumberg (pictured left) wrote[1] : "In patients undergoing hip replacement or spine surgery, the postoperative infection rate with allogeneic blood transfusion appears to be seven to ten-fold higher than with autologous blood or no transfusion."

Along with a greater incidence of postoperative infection, more rapid progression of HIV, the activation of latent viruses, prolonged postoperative ventilatory support and poor wound healing, inevitably go higher medical and hospitalization costs.

Additionally, the negative effects of transfusions appear to be dose-dependent. That is, they increase with the amount of blood given. Every additional unit of blood transfused presents a greater risk of infection, prolonged hospitalization and higher costs. A recent study estimated that the risk of postoperative infection or pneumonia increased by 6% for each unit transfused. Two studies, one in New York and the other in Denmark, calculated an incremental postoperative cost due to transfusion of US$1,000 to US$2,000 for each unit of allogeneic blood given. A clear example of its effect on hospital stay shows in Professor Blumberg's accompanying chart. Studies analyzing this have made allowance in their calculations for confounding factors such as age of patient, sex, severity of illness, complexity of operation, and so on.

Investigating the association of allogeneic blood with serious postoperative infection and pneumonia, Professor Jeffrey Carson and colleagues reviewed 9,598 consecutive operations to repair broken hips in patients over 60 years of age. Their study was published in the July 1999 issue of the medical journal *Transfusion*. Information was collected from 20 hospitals on operations performed between 1983 and 1993. Analysis

Average length of hospital stay by number of allogeneic blood units transfused in patients undergoing hip replacement surgery

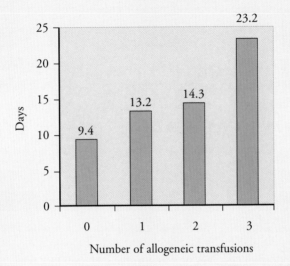

Postoperative infection is one of the major causes of longer hospital stays. Postoperative infection rates appear to increase with the number of units transfused. The above chart shows the results of a study conducted by Professor Neil Blumberg and colleagues showing the average length of hospital stay by the number of units of allogeneic blood transfused in patients having hip replacement surgery. All patients donated their own blood prior to surgery and then either did or did not receive allogeneic blood. Chart reprinted with permission. Blumberg N. Allogeneic Transfusion and Infection: Economic and Clinical Implications. *Seminars in Hematology.* July 1997;34(3) (suppl 2):34-40.

of the data revealed that 58% of the patients were transfused and that there was a dose-response relationship for serious infection. The risk of infection increased with each unit transfused. Overall, 4.6% of the patients suffered a serious postoperative infection. They concluded that there was a 35% greater risk of serious bacterial infection and a 52% greater risk of pneumonia associated with blood transfusion.

They also calculated the extra cost of treating those infections. On average, infection incurred an extra cost of $14,000 for each patient. Additionally, 28.8% of those with serious infections died while in hospital. Consequently, Carson's group concluded: "The risk of bacterial infection may be the most common life-threatening adverse effect of allogeneic blood transfusion."

In the context of this book, their recommendations following the study are noteworthy. One was that more efforts must be directed towards reducing allogeneic blood; another, that the exploration of alternatives must continue.

The immune suppression effect of transfusion may also contribute to a poorer outcome in cancer surgery. While still a controversial area under investigation, the weight of studies indicates that if a patient is transfused while undergoing surgery, the cancer will recur sooner and the survival time will be reduced. This has been shown in reports for most types of cancer surgery, including lung, head, neck, liver, prostate, uterus and genital tract, colon, stomach and the extremities.

These studies have shown that cancer patients who are transfused have up to almost four times greater risk of recurrence and/or death compared with patients who are not transfused.[2]

Professor Blumberg and a colleague, writing in *The American Journal of Medicine* in 1996, suggested the scientific evidence for this was as strong as early data linking smoking to cardiovascular disease and cancer. More recently, he suggested inadequate attention had been given to this potential effect of transfusion which, he said, had significant implications for public health, including increased patient deaths and costs.

Blumberg and his associate went on to conduct a theoretical analysis from medical literature. This sought to estimate the potential death rate from postoperative infection and cancer recurrence caused by immune suppression from transfusion. They concluded that a very conservative figure would be 215 deaths a year if only 1% of the immune suppression effect caused postoperative infection and cancer recurrence. However, they estimated deaths could be as many as 21,500 if the effect was 100% causal. From their research they assessed that more than 90% was causal. This compared with an estimated 30 deaths a year from HIV-1 through transfusion.

Professor Blumberg reinforced their original findings when he noted[3]: "Our estimates suggest that the death rate from immunomodulation (immune suppression) may exceed the death rate due to all other transfusion risks combined."

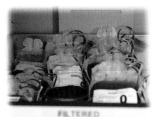

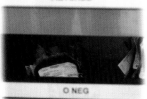

While it is not known which of the blood components are responsible, recent investigations suggest that white cells in the transfused blood may contribute to this immune suppression, along with a number of other short-term and long-term transfusion complications. Blood products, including whole blood, red blood cells and platelets, contain large numbers of leukocytes, or white blood cells. Special filters have been developed, called *leukocyte depletion filters*, which are able to remove most of the white cells from stored blood and appear to reduce or delay some transfusion problems.

A study conducted by Dr Paul Tartter and colleagues from New York's Mount Sinai Medical Center examined patients undergoing gastrointestinal (stomach and intestine) surgery. They compared the rates of infection, length of hospital stay and cost among those receiving conventional blood transfusions, filtered transfusions (leukodepleted blood) and those receiving no transfusions.

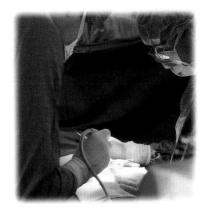

Of the 221 patients studied, 27% were transfused. Avoidance of transfusion was not the objective of the study. As a result, multiple blood conservation measures were not integrated into the management plan for the patients under investigation. Infections occurred in 11% of those receiving no blood, in 16% of those receiving filtered blood and in 44% receiving unfiltered blood. The average hospital stay after surgery was nine days in the untransfused group, 12 in the filtered group and 18 in the unfiltered group. Hospital charges were also markedly different — US$19,132, US$33,954 and US$41,002, respectively.

White cells in blood products are also believed to be responsible for some of the other transfusion complications. For these reasons, some transfusion services have begun leukodepletion of all their blood before storage with the aim of reducing these adverse effects and risks.

A number of medical experts have emphasized that immune suppression is the most urgent issue concerning blood transfusion today.

The passage of time seems to have imparted considerable weight to Dr John Spratt's comment in *The American Journal of Surgery* back in 1986 when he wrote "the cancer surgeon may need to become a bloodless surgeon."

The negative effects of immune suppression can be summarized thus:

- Earlier cancer recurrence and decreased survival
- Greater incidence of postoperative infection
- Prolonged postoperative ventilatory support
- Poor wound healing
- More antibiotic therapy
- Lengthier hospital stays
- More rapid progression of HIV/AIDS
- Activation of latent viruses

Clearly, concern over possible infection and cancer recurrence from transfusion-induced immune suppression adds to the desirability of bloodless surgery.

Effects of Storage on Blood

Blood stored for transfusion is a different product from that which travels around our body. Blood is a living biological product which, once removed from the body, begins to break down and change chemically and physically. This is despite the addition of anticoagulants and preservatives and being stored at about 4° C. The deterioration that takes place in storage is sometimes referred to as the *storage lesion.*

In Chapter 2, we described how red blood cells need to fold and squeeze through very small capillaries to deliver their load of oxygen to the cells in the tissue. In storage, however, the red cells change shape from discs to spheres and the membranes lose their flexibility and become more rigid. So they are less able to squeeze through the microcirculation.

SLIDE 1

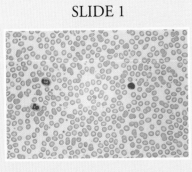

Normal blood.

SLIDE 2

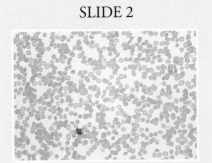

Red blood cells that have been stored for three weeks. The cells have changed shape, their membranes have become more rigid and cells have clumped together. Cell membrane breakdown is also evident.

The substance (2,3-DPG) that regulates the hemoglobin's ability to release its load of oxygen is lost in storage. The oxygen is bound more tightly and isn't let go as easily to the tissues. Oxygen released by other normal cells can even be "grabbed" by this hemoglobin. As a result, the transfused blood intended to provide *additional* oxygen to the patient at a time of critical need may, in fact, be robbing the patient of *existing* oxygen, worsening the outcome.

The blood cells and other components also begin to break down. Some of the cells rupture, spilling out their contents. Clumps then form, made up of these cell fragments, other debris, fibrin, platelets and white cells which, along with the formation of small clots, further impair blood flow. The chemical balance also changes in the blood stored in the plastic bag. Moreover, because the blood is exposed to foreign surfaces and additive substances, its activated white blood cells and other immune responses create undesirable reactions when transfused into another person. This is not surprising, since it is the precise defence role that the white cells are programmed to undertake.

Little wonder that, with all these changes, such blood when transfused can be detrimental, especially to a critically ill patient.

In a seminal study of transfusion policies in intensive care unit patients, Dr Paul Hébert and his colleagues demonstrated that acutely ill patients had an increased risk of dying if they were transfused liberally. This study highlights the negative impact of transfusing stored blood (see Chapter 4).

These harmful effects appear to increase with each day of storage. In the July 1999 issue of *Transfusion*, Dr E. C. Vamvakas, of the New York University Medical Center's Transfusion Services, published his study of heart surgery patients, establishing an association between the length of storage and the development of postoperative infection. Dr Vamvakas calculated the risk of pneumonia rose by 1% per day of increase in the mean storage time of the transfused red blood cells.

It has also been suggested that the release of various bioactive substances during storage may contribute to the immune suppression effect.

The storage lesion problems can be summarized thus:
- Red cells become less flexible and change shape
- Loss of the compound 2,3-DPG results in oxygen binding more tightly to hemoglobin and not being released as easily to the tissues
- Elevated levels of sodium, glucose, potassium, ammonium and lactic acid
- Changes from slightly alkaline to slightly acidic
- Rupture of some red cells
- Red cell survival shortened
- Debris and breakdown products
- Formation of small clots
- Formation of clumps of debris and other cells (microaggregates)
- Activation of white cells
- Release of various bioactive substances
- Loss of clotting factors and platelets
- Toxicity from the additive substances
- Toxicity from the plasticizers in the bag

Note: These changes also take place in stored autologous (one's own) blood.

Other Reactions

Blood is an organ and a transfusion is essentially an organ transplant. Everyone's blood is highly individual and a transfusion is subject to similar complications and reactions as other organ transplants. Consequently, the body can react, sometimes severely, when foreign blood is introduced.

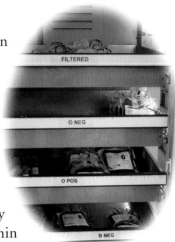

Adverse transfusion reactions are divided into two categories: immune and non-immune. Both may be immediate or delayed, occurring either within minutes to hours of the transfusion, or several days or even months later.

Immune reactions are extremely difficult to avoid because of the highly individual nature of each person's blood. In the previous chapter we discussed Landsteiner's discovery of the major blood groups. He distinguished one grouping from another by the presence of specific proteins, called antigens, on the surface of the red blood cells. As a result of this research, Landsteiner and others were able to divide people into four main blood categories: those with one type of antigen into group A, those with another into B, those with neither A nor B into O and those with both A and B antigens as AB.

In everyone's plasma are naturally occurring antibodies. These react against foreign antigens; that is, antigens not normally present on a particular person's red blood cells. For example, those with type A blood (A antigens on the red blood cell's surface) will have anti-B antibodies in their plasma which will attack type B blood. This ABO system is the most clinically significant blood grouping and, should these types be wrongly transfused, they cause serious and sometimes fatal reactions.

Transfusion medicine experts underline the gravity of this problem.

In 1994, a leading British medical journal[4] reported that both medical and public opinion at that time would probably rank HIV transmission as the prime complication of donor blood. In fact, said the report, the single biggest cause of mortality remained transfusion of the wrong pack of blood, potentially resulting in major ABO incompatibility. The study went on to note: "There is no formal reporting system for either major transfusion errors or 'near miss' events, but a recent survey suggests that the risk of such an incident is approximately 1 in every 30,000 units transfused."

Four years on, doctors Arnold C. Y. Chen and Jeffrey L. Carson[5], reported: "Unfortunately, a significant proportion of fatal transfusion reactions occur during surgery, where the reaction may be more difficult to diagnose. Symptoms of a transfusion reaction may either be masked by general anaesthesia or may be non-specific and attributed to other causes."

The complex nature of the blood system and its composition goes far beyond those main groupings. Since Landsteiner's time, hundreds of blood types have been discovered. Antigens are also present on white blood cells, platelets and in plasma. In addition to naturally occurring antibodies to these antigens, the body can also develop antibodies in response to being exposed to certain antigens (alloimmunization). For example, this can occur after a previous transfusion or pregnancy.

In fact, there are so many antigen, antibody and protein combinations that it is highly unlikely any two individuals would have identical, perfectly matched blood, the possible exceptions being identical twins. Despite careful ABO grouping of blood and careful pre-transfusion cross-matching of the donor units with the patient's blood to detect other antigens and antibodies, reactions still occur.

As indicated, these can vary from mild to life-threatening. They can create chills and fevers, cause low blood pressure and breathing difficulties, create severe allergic reactions, affect kidney, lung and other body functions and, at worst, cause death.

There are other transfusion complications such as volume overload, iron overload, coagulation disturbances, metabolic complications, bacterial contamination during blood collecting and processing and so on. A more comprehensive list of these along with the estimated risk and why they occur, appears in Appendix I (see p.148).

Given the very real complications and risks of receiving stored blood from another person, it is logical to ask: Is there another way?

"Blood transfusion has never been as safe a procedure as most patients and clinicians have thought, with a plethora of potential complications and new ones still being recognized. There is persisting pressure from society driven by a perceived need to further minimize or abolish the infectious complications of allogeneic transfusion. The clinician has a clear role in achieving this end by avoiding allogeneic transfusion whenever possible."

Dr. James Isbister
Risk Management in Transfusion Medicine. *Transfusion Medicine Reviews* 1996;10(3):183-202.

"Even if known infectious complications could be eliminated, transfusion of [allogeneic blood products] will never be a totally safe procedure. New transfusion-related complications, the magnitude of which is unknown, . . . have emerged recently. . . Other, as yet unidentified, pathogens will undoubtedly be transmitted by [allogeneic blood] in the future."

Dr. J. F. Hardy, Blood products: when to use them and how to avoid them. *Canadian Journal of Anaesthesia* 1994;41(Suppl Pt 2):R52-R61.

"If one approached regulatory authorities today with a new product with the safety profile of human red cells, it probably would not be approved for clinical use."

Robert Winslow, Professor of Medicine, University of California, San Diego, as reported in the May 18, 1996 cover story in Canada's *The Globe and Mail* newspaper, "Alternatives to transfusion grow popular."

[1] Blumberg, Neil; MD; Professor of Pathology and Laboratory Medicine, Director of Transfusion Medicine Unit, University of Rochester School of Medicine and Dentistry, Rochester NY. Allogeneic Transfusion and Infection: Economic and Clinical Implications. *Seminars in Hematology* 1997; 34(3) (suppl. 2): 34-40

[2] The effect of suppressing the immune system does have some unexpected benefits in certain circumstances. These include a lesser incidence of organ transplant rejection, reduced recurrent spontaneous abortion and disease reduction in rheumatoid arthritis and Crohn's disease (chronic inflammation of the intestine). The beneficial effects appear to be the result of elements in the transfused blood altering the immune system's reaction to foreign organs (transplant and fetus) and some inflammation diseases (rheumatoid arthritis and Crohn's disease).

[3] Blumberg, Neil, MD; Allogeneic Transfusion and Infection: Economic and Clinical Implications. *Seminars in Hematology* 1997;34(3) (suppl. 2):34-40

[4] Williams L. Homologous Blood Transfusion: The Risk and Alternatives. *British Journal of Haematology* 1994;88(3);451-458

[5] Chen, Dr Arnold C.Y.; Carson, Dr Jeffrey L.; Perioperative management of anaemia, *British Journal of Anaesthesia* 1998;81(Suppl.1):20-24

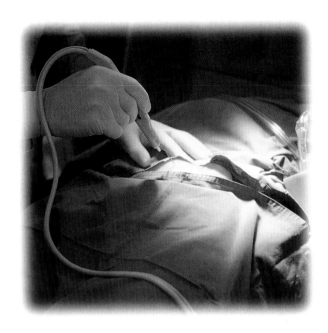

CHAPTER 4

YOUR BODY, YOUR CHOICE

An Alternative, or the Only Way to Go?

According to France's eminent Professor Bernard Glorion, the benefits of transfusion appeared to outweigh all disadvantages . . . that is, until that critical point when evidence to the contrary became unmistakably clear.

Speaking at a Paris international symposium on bloodless surgery in 1996, Professor Glorion emphasized that the indisputable risks of transfusion and the associated medical, economic and human consequences were such that they now simply had to be considered. Glorion, Professeur des Universites and President du Conseil national de l'Ordre national des medecins, indicated that the medical world was forced to respond. Every surgical team had to face the thorny problems posed by blood transfusion and seek ways of performing bloodless surgery.

The Professor noted that bloodless surgery, despite its undoubted good sense, was the very opposite to what the medical profession had been accustomed.

So, should the profession be looking merely for an alternative; a system that functions only on occasional demands and is practiced by a select group of devotees to a cause? Or are we poised on the threshold of a revolutionary approach, another dimension for medicine, which departs from unfounded tradition and demands new standards in health care?

Leading California-based heart surgeon, Manuel Estioko[1], speaking in his Good Samaritan Hospital clinic in Los Angeles, California, recently, was adamant that what he and his colleagues preferred to call the "transfusion-free" approach to surgery should never be regarded as a mere alternative.

"'Alternative' is an inferior word," said Dr Estioko who is founder and Medical Director of the Transfusion-Free Medicine and Surgery Center at Good

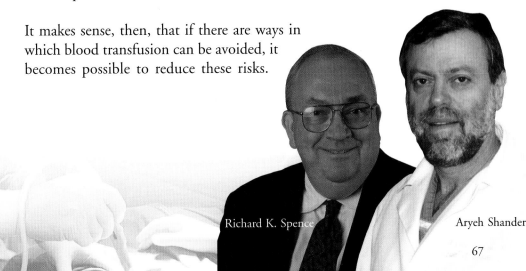

Samaritan. "Transfusion-free surgery is superior to mainstream medicine and there should be no alternative to it." He predicted that medicine had no other route to take in the years ahead. Science and society would simply insist on it.

While Manuel Estioko (pictured left) in California, Richard K. Spence[2] in Alabama, Aryeh Shander[3] in New York (pictured below) and Donat Spahn[4] in Zurich are at the forefront of this challenging new direction, there remain critics and detractors. Still, the mounting ground-swell of support for bloodless surgery throughout the world is undeniable. The tide is turning inexorably.

Statistics on surgical survival rates provide a case in point. Survival rates tend to go down with more blood transfused. This was actually recognised as early as the 1980s. A Canadian study published in *The Canadian Journal of Surgery*, 1988, reported that in patients with rectal cancer, the 10-year survival rate was 82% for patients with no blood transfusion. In contrast, there was a 53% survival rate for patients who had received 1 to 5 units of blood, 31% for those with 6 to 10 units and 14% for those who had been given more than 10 units. Several recent studies have similarly indicated that multiple red blood cell transfusions are associated with increased risk of morbidity and mortality.

These are sobering statistics, defying and denying the perceptions held for many years that "blood transfusion = life", "no blood transfusion = death," and that there are no other options. These equations are, quite clearly, not that simple.

It makes sense, then, that if there are ways in which blood transfusion can be avoided, it becomes possible to reduce these risks.

Richard K. Spence

Aryeh Shander

67

This, in itself, can only be advantageous. Could it be like the English fairytale experience of Winnie-the-Pooh who kept bumping his head as Christopher Robin dragged him downstairs backwards by his heels? "It is, as far as he knows, the only way of coming downstairs, but sometimes he feels that there really is another way, if only he could stop bumping for a moment and think of it."

Bloodless surgery offers "another way." It focuses on many methods and techniques designed to avoid exposure to blood. For the patient, the good news is there is increasing clinical evidence not only of reduced risks, but also of a whole range of positive benefits.

Six Good Reasons for Wanting Bloodless Surgery

Let's look at some of the positive benefits of this "other way" approach:

- You avoid the potential risks of contracting disease.
- You avoid a host of transfusion reactions and possible complications.
- You enhance your chances of quicker recovery after an operation.
- You generally can expect to spend fewer bed-days in hospital, with consequently lower hospital and medical costs.
- If you have surgery for cancer, chances for your long-term survival are likely to be improved.
- You reduce the risk of getting an infection after an operation and are thereby less likely to need antibiotic therapy with its attendant risks and complications.

However, bloodless or transfusion-free surgery, while a growing field of medicine that crosses all disciplines, is not standard practice yet. You are not going to get it routinely when you discuss the need for surgery with your doctor. You may have to seek out specialists who practice it.

What is important to understand is that the bloodless way is an option open to everyone wanting to avoid the risks of allogeneic blood. More and more people are recognizing its advantages, placing pressure on medicine and science to react to consumer demand. Increasingly, in advanced communities, people want to have more say in their medical management. They want to be consulted and thoroughly briefed so they can weigh risks and benefits and make informed decisions. It is important to understand that *informed choice* is a recognized legal cornerstone granting patients the right of bodily self-determination.

Not surprisingly, bloodless surgery techniques have their greatest application in operations carrying the risk of significant blood loss. The many types of heart and vascular surgery, along with orthopedic surgery, where operations such as hip and knee replacements have become increasingly common, are either 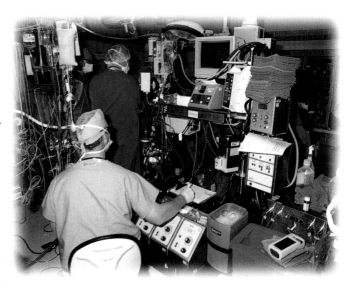 traditionally major blood loss procedures or, at least, have the potential to be very "bloody." Then there is cancer surgery where some of the major procedures, such as abdominal and bone tumor surgery, likewise carry a similar degree of risk.

These and other surgical procedures are all ideal candidates for the application of bloodless surgery techniques. At very least, these will help minimize the amount of blood used, thereby reducing the number of donors to whom the patient is exposed and, consequently, the risk of contaminated blood.

There is also considerable concern these days about the overuse of antibiotics and their side-effects. As with blood itself, unnecessary use can be dangerous.

Internationally, the message grows stronger by the day: the goal for surgeons must be to reduce the use of blood transfusion. Accompanying this call is an expanding new list of expressions — *blood conservation, blood management, non-blood management, transfusion-free, transfusion alternatives, hemovigilance* and so on.

Conferences Set New Guidelines

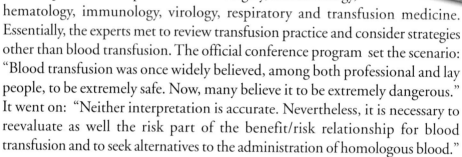

Consensus conferences offer the opportunities for experts in all the fields of medicine around the world to get together and review practice. The conferences are also designed to educate and keep everyone tuned in to the most recent developments in ongoing research.

In 1988, the US National Institute of Health (NIH) convened an important consensus conference on blood transfusion for world experts in the respective fields of surgery, anesthesiology, hematology, immunology, virology, respiratory and transfusion medicine. Essentially, the experts met to review transfusion practice and consider strategies other than blood transfusion. The official conference program set the scenario: "Blood transfusion was once widely believed, among both professional and lay people, to be extremely safe. Now, many believe it to be extremely dangerous." It went on: "Neither interpretation is accurate. Nevertheless, it is necessary to reevaluate as well the risk part of the benefit/risk relationship for blood transfusion and to seek alternatives to the administration of homologous blood."

One speaker, Howard Zauder, a professor of anesthesiology, emphasized that certain long-standing transfusion practice was based more on tradition than clinical and scientific evidence. He told his colleagues: "The etiology of the requirement that a patient have 10 grams of hemoglobin prior to receiving an anesthetic is cloaked in tradition, shrouded in obscurity, and unsubstantiated by clinical or experimental evidence."

In the same context, the subsequent report on the NIH conference, published in *The Journal of the American Medical Association*, admitted that medical literature was "remarkable for the absence of carefully controlled, randomized trials that would permit definitive conclusions regarding perioperative transfusion practice."

Also in 1988, the *Report of the Presidential Commission on the Human Immunodeficiency Virus Epidemic* said flatly that many doctors and hospitals did not have an adequate understanding of the availability of alternatives to traditional transfusion therapy. The report recommended that health care facilities adopt all reasonable strategies to avoid allogeneic transfusion, including predeposited autologous transfusions, hemodilution techniques, intraoperative autologous transfusions, and postoperative collection. It went on to advocate aggressive in-service training for health care staff, particularly for blood banking and transfusion services personnel.

These quite extraordinary acknowledgements would gather further momentum. In 1992, the American College of Physicians sponsored a comprehensive review of transfusion practice that ultimately revealed there had never been controlled clinical trials of blood transfusion.

As with the 1988 conference report, the American College of Physicians' review, four years later, concluded there was need for more research. The impact of these two important documents was to encourage development of what were already being regarded as promising alternatives to transfusion. The need for greater doctor education was also expressed strongly at the time.

In the following years, a number of other medical groups conducted consensus conferences and issued transfusion practice guidelines.

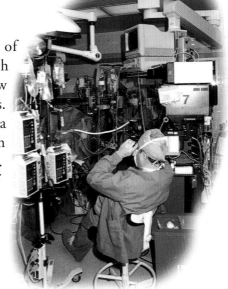

In March, 1996, the American Society of Anesthesiologists published the research results of a task force formed to review transfusion practice and set new guidelines. They concluded there was still a lack of data from randomized studies to establish evidence-based practice guidelines. Alternative strategies were seen as a way of reducing exposure to blood and its potential adverse effects. It was recommended there be a more discriminating approach to transfusion based on patient symptoms rather than traditional transfusion practice.

Despite differing opinions and practices among doctors, quiet progress was being made. By August 1996, *The American Journal of Medicine* was reporting on the changes that had occurred in the use of blood transfusion over the previous decade. The application of multiple alternatives had seen a steady decrease in the amount of blood transfused. Many heart surgery patients, who previously received 20 to 30 units of blood, were now given no blood at all. Many traditionally high blood-loss orthopedic surgery patients received no blood either. One institution reported 90% of its heart bypass operations were now being done without blood.

This developing new understanding of blood underscored emerging new attitudes by the medical world towards transfusions and the dawning realization that better methods and approaches might offer safer and more cost-effective outcomes. The tide may have ebbed, but it was yet to turn. An audit of hospitals found that their transfusion practices were still extremely varied. It indicated that too many blood transfusions were still inappropriate, and highlighted there was yet much to be done and much to be learned.

Canadian Study's Dramatic Results

The results of a Canadian study reported in a 1999 issue of *The New England Journal of Medicine* showed that tolerating anemia and minimizing or avoiding blood transfusion in critically ill patients actually saved lives. The study dealt with transfusion requirements in critical care and its findings were obviously contrary to the widely held assumption that such patients should be "topped up" to an arbitrary level. In other words, it showed that "less is more." This appears to have been the first-ever large clinical trial examining the effectiveness of blood transfusion practices on critically ill patients.

The study, known as TRICC – an acronym for Transfusion Requirements in Critical Care – was headed by Dr Paul Hébert, a critical care specialist at Ottawa General Hospital. It involved 838 patients at 25 Canadian hospitals, all of whom were also suffering from anemia. They were divided into two groups. Half (420) were assigned to a liberal transfusion strategy. This meant they would be transfused if their hemoglobin dropped below 10 g/dL, the traditional transfusion trigger. Furthermore, they would be maintained between 10 g/dL and 12 g/dL. The other half (418) were assigned to a restrictive policy. They would be transfused only if their hemoglobin dropped below 7 g/dL. If they received blood, they would be maintained between 7 g/dL and 9 g/dL. As it happened, because of this restrictive policy, 33% of the latter group received no blood at all. Doctors then compared the death rates and organ dysfunction in these patients to assess the effects of the two strategies.

The results were dramatic. (See the summary below.) Overall, the mortality rate during hospitalization was higher in the liberal strategy group (28.1% versus 22.2%), as was the incidence of heart and lung complications and organ dysfunction. Of particular interest, there were comparatively more deaths in the liberal group's patients who were less acutely ill (one additional death for every 13 patients). Similarly, there were more deaths in the liberal group's under 55 years of age category (one additional death for every 14 patients).

Table. Summary of the TRICC study results

	Mortality rate in %		
	Liberal transfusion strategy	Restrictive transfusion strategy	P Value
30 Days	23.3	18.7	0.11
60 Days	26.5	22.7	0.23
During ICU stay	16.2	13.9	0.29
During hospital stay	28.1	22.2	0.05
Those aged less than 55 years	13.0	5.7	0.02
Those less acutely ill	16.1	8.7	0.03
Those with significant heart disease	22.9	20.5	0.69

	Average length of stay in days		
	Liberal transfusion strategy	Restrictive transfusion strategy	P Value
In ICU	11.5	11.0	0.53
In hospital	35.5	34.8	0.58

Chart compiled from data in Hébert PC. et al. A Multicenter, Randomized, Controlled Clinical Trial of Transfusion Requirements in Critical Care. *The New England Journal of Medicine* 1999; 340(6):409-17. For those familiar with statistics, the P value has been included.

Dr Hébert and his colleagues concluded that the increased mortality and complications may have resulted from the storage lesion, the physical and biochemical changes that take place in stored blood. Others have suggested the immunosuppressive effect of allogeneic blood may have played a part. In a subsequent newspaper report, Dr Hébert observed: "We've been transfusing blood for 50 years and no one's ever bothered to find out how much to give. Now we know it's safe to transfuse less."

An editorial on the Canadian study published in *The New England Journal of Medicine* commented that "transfusion practice is a striking example of how some patterns of treatment in critical care may have been set prematurely." By challenging current practice, said the journal, Dr Hébert and other investigators had made it clear that a single threshold for transfusion in all patients was not appropriate. It also stated that if the restrictive transfusion strategy was widely adopted, there would be "laudable" cost savings and conservation of blood.

Reduced Costs and Hospital Stays

In 1998, Dr Todd Rosengart[5] and his colleagues from the New York Hospital's Cornell University Medical Center published the results of a multimodality[6] blood conservation program. They had developed the program to minimize allogeneic transfusions in heart surgery. Initially, it was applied successfully to 50 patients who, for religious reasons, did not want blood transfusions. The results were published in the June, 1998, issue of the *Journal of the American College of Surgeons.*

Operations included coronary artery bypass graft (CABG), valve replacement, valve and bypass operations, multiple valve replacements and reoperations; in short, a whole range of complex heart surgery. When compared with a group of patients with matched diagnosis, in whom the multimodality "bloodless" strategy was not applied, it was evident that bloodless surgery patients tended to have shorter lengths of stay in hospital and one group had reduced costs.

The results were so encouraging it was decided to extend the bloodless approach to their general heart surgery patients. Refinements were made to the methods applied. Instead of using all strategies for every patient, they were used selectively according to the individual patient's needs. A study was made of its efficacy and cost-effectiveness and published in the journal *Annals of Thoracic Surgery,* 1998.

Over three months Rosengart and his team successfully carried out 100 consecutive heart operations (CABG) without using allogeneic blood. They then compared these results with the records of similar patients whose operations were performed without the multimodality approach and where allogeneic blood transfusions had been used. Results showed that time on the ventilator after surgery was reduced significantly in the bloodless group (18 hours against 22 hours). Although not statistically significant, the average length of stay in intensive care was also shorter (42 hours against 44 hours). Additionally, postoperative hospital stay was less (7.4 days against 8.9 days). When compared with another group of patients matched by diagnosis and operated on before the multimodality approach, the average costs for the bloodless surgery group were 10 – 24% less and length of stay was 16 – 26% less.

The notable results of another study, this time of 487 consecutive patients undergoing cancer surgery, were published in the February, 1998 issue of *Archives of Pathology and Laboratory Medicine.* They showed that for every unit of blood transfused, the hospital stay increased by 1.3% and costs by 2%. This was even after allowing for variables in severity of illness, difficulty of operation and other factors. In real terms, this meant the length of hospitalization for these patients varied from 16.7 days for the transfused group to 10.3 days for the untransfused. The hospital charges for each patient in the two groups amounted to US$28,101 and US$15,978 respectively.

Addressing a conference in Cleveland in 1995, Dr David Rosencrantz, Medical Director of Bloodless Medicine and Surgery at Good Samaritan Hospital in Portland, Oregon, reported his bloodless surgery patients spent a similar time in the postoperative recovery room to patients who had been transfused. However, they spent a slightly shorter time in intensive care and were out of hospital on average one day sooner.

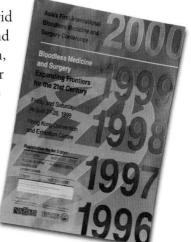

At the 1999 International Bloodless Medicine and Surgery Conference in Hong Kong, data were presented from the 1997 annual report of the Center for Bloodless Medicine and Surgery at the University of Miami/Jackson Memorial Medical Center. For that year the average length of stay was 5.6 days for those enrolled in the bloodless surgery program. This compared with 6.6 days for those not enrolled. The resulting saving in costs over the year amounted to US$691,710.24.

Meanwhile, a Canadian hospital's experience with liver transplantation has confirmed that reducing blood use from between 20 to 100 units a transplant to an average of 6 units decreased hospital stay days from an average of three weeks to 10 days.

The surgical techniques themselves in bloodless surgery offer direct advantages to the patient's recovery. A basic principle of bloodless surgical technique is careful, gentle tissue handling to reduce blood loss, as you will discover in the next chapter. There is less trauma to the tissue and so reduced release of the enzymes and chemicals that cause pain. In addition, less bleeding into the tissue may decrease the incidence of postoperative infection. The combined effects mean, on average, fewer postoperative complications and better recovery.

Less bleeding into the operative site also means a clearer field of work for the surgeon. He or she can then work with greater speed and assurance. Some reports have suggested that this, in turn, brings about a more complete job, shortening the operation time and reducing the period the person is exposed to anesthetic.

Blood: A Finite Resource

A major consideration of the whole blood question is the limited supply and the increasing costs associated with collecting, screening and testing.

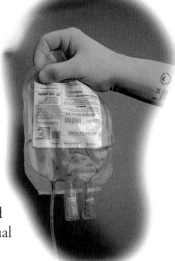

Blood is no longer seen as an infinite resource. Transfusion services worldwide are finding it increasingly difficult to maintain supplies, let alone expand them. They predict this will become more critical as aging segments of populations expand and require more complex surgery. Experts predict an annual four million unit deficit by the year 2030. This presents a two-fold frustration for transfusion services which, while trying to cope with the higher demand, also know that blood is being used inappropriately on many patients who don't really need it. Studies estimate that as many as 66% of all transfusions administered may be unnecessary, with the knock-on effect being further pressure on the availability of sufficient blood for patients considered most in need of it.

There are several reasons for dwindling blood supplies. One is that as transfusion services apply increasingly stringent tests to improve safety levels, potential donors are correspondingly being screened out. According to a 1999 article in *The New England Journal of Medicine*, half-a-million blood donors are disqualified each year in the US because of positive test results. People are also becoming more reluctant to donate blood in an environment that has drawn so much adverse publicity. A recent report in Britain noted a decreasing "altruistic spirit of the community" towards being donors.

The Real Cost is Getting Higher

In many countries unpaid volunteer donors supply blood. In turn, their donated blood is frequently provided free of charge to hospitals. But everybody knows 'there is no such thing as a free lunch.' Someone, somewhere, has to pay. More often than not, it finally comes down to the taxpayer's responsibility. The job of collecting blood, screening donors and testing, storing and transporting blood happens to be a costly exercise. Every time a new virus comes along, a new test is needed. Inevitably, that means additional costs. For example, in 1995, when the American FDA (Food and Drug Administration) decided to use a new HIV blood test, it was estimated it would cost between US$60 million to US$100 million a year.

How much does a unit of blood cost? That depends on what you count. If you just count collecting, screening, testing and supplying blood, estimates vary from US$100 to US$300 a unit.

However, a 1991 American assessment estimated that if one considers direct expenses, costs of treating complications of transfusions and indirect outlays, each unit of blood comes at an estimated US$1,332. Even so, it appears what has not been taken into account in this appraisal is the additional cost of a liver transplantation resulting from a transfusion complication. Most liver transplants in the US today are the consequence of hepatitis C and can cost an average $300,000 each. On top of this is an additional $25,000 for medications every year for each patient for the rest of his or her life. An estimated 5,000 liver transplants are performed every year in the US. If the liver disease was caused by a blood transfusion, that should rightly go on the "blood bill" over and above the US$1,332 for each unit.

What, then, is the economic cost to society through lost productivity of those people with HIV or hepatitis C? Add to this the bills associated with immune suppression discussed in the previous chapter. Additionally, one must surely take into account the financial impact on patients and families faced with cancer recurrence.

Postoperative fever is a common reaction following transfusion. Investigating and treating this reaction costs money. It often involves a chest x-ray, urine analysis, blood tests, administering antibiotics and an increased stay in hospital. Dr Paul Potter, of the Cleveland Clinic Foundation, calculates that treating just this one transfusion complication delivers an annual bill of some US$4.6 billion to the American health system.

Professor Neil Blumberg has concluded that allogeneic blood transfusion adds incremental costs to patient care at a rate of US$1,000 to US$1,500 per unit. The extra cost results from increased postoperative infection due to immune suppression, increased use of antibiotics and prolonged hospital stay.

All this shows how difficult it is to establish realistically what blood actually costs the community. The unit price obviously is very high, indeed. Equally obvious, bloodless surgery strategies can help substantially reduce this cost.

Litigation — A Growing Concern

Liability in connection with transfusion is an ever present and growing concern for clinicians. Doctors have a duty to inform their patients of the risks or side-effects of any proposed treatment. They must also acquaint their patients with any alternative means of available treatment. Some legal opinion maintains that doctors and hospitals who fail to inform their patients about the risks of blood transfusion and neglect to offer alternatives, could be liable for complications that arise.

Dr Paul Tartter wrote in the *Journal of Intensive Care Medicine*: "Million-dollar lawsuits for acquired immunodeficiency syndrome contracted by patients given unnecessary blood are being won by the plaintiffs, whereas lawsuits for wrongful death because blood was withheld are rare." Another prominent US surgeon, Dr Ciril Godec, said that the benefit of transfusion was so questionable that many surgeons had adopted a philosophy of "transfusion avoidance", not only for medical but also for legal reasons.

Some American states, like California (The Paul Gann Blood Safety Act), New Jersey (The Blood Safety Act of 1991) and Texas, have enacted legislation that requires the doctor to inform each patient who may face the possibility of receiving allogeneic blood of the risks and benefits — and of the alternatives available. These discussions are documented in their medical records and some acts require that written informed consent to a blood transfusion must be obtained from the patient.

Published impact studies reveal that such legislation, requiring informed consent to the administration of blood and blood products, has had a positive effect on the transfusion practices of doctors.

> *"I believe that diseases that are going to be the subject of lawsuits in the next century are being transfused in your patients today."*

Dr Benjamin Reichstein, Director of Surgery, Columbia St Vincent Charity Hospital, Cleveland, Ohio.

> *"A typical transfusion malpractice case would be one in which the transfusion is shown to have been unnecessary or improperly administered – or one in which a practitioner failed to provide reasonable and prudent alternatives."*

Edward B. Goldman JD, University of Michigan Medical Center. Legal Considerations for Allogeneic Blood Transfusion. *The American Journal of Surgery* 1995;170(suppl 6A):27S-31S.

Patients and the Right to Decide

In most countries, courts have affirmed the principle of "patient autonomy." This is protected through the "informed consent" process. It involves the rights of the informed patient to bodily integrity and self-determination. Inherent, here, is the right to weigh treatment options and their respective risks and benefits and make decisions about medical procedures and what is done to their body. Ultimately, this involves the fundamental right to choose between different types of treatment or even to refuse one recommended by a doctor.

The principle of informed consent received international attention following the Nuremberg Trials. Details of atrocities forced on people in concentration camps during World War II in the name of medical science led to serious concerns about treatments being performed on non-consenting individuals. Out of this has grown a real emphasis on patient autonomy and informed consent. The book, *An American Civil Liberties Union Handbook: The Rights of Patients*, describes informed consent as "the most important legal doctrine in both the doctor-patient relationship and treatment in health care facilities."

Accordingly, many health organizations and hospitals have developed charters or statements of patient rights. In 1993, a working party of the National Health and Medical Research Council of Australia published guidelines for doctors on how best to provide information to patients. The aim was to "reflect the common law right of legally competent patients to make their own decisions about medical treatment, and their right to grant, withhold or withdraw consent before or during examination or treatment." The guidelines added: "The community recognizes that patients are entitled to make their own decisions. In order to do so, they must have enough information about their condition, investigation options, treatment options, benefits, possible adverse effects of investigations or treatment, and the likely result if treatment is not undertaken."

Most surgical procedures have their own risks or side-effects. Patients therefore have to weigh the risks and the benefits. For example, in treating cancer, a doctor may offer the options of surgery, chemotherapy or radiation therapy. The doctor may suggest that, in this particular case, surgery has an expected 80% success rate, chemotherapy 85% and radiation therapy 78%. These figures are just examples and do not reflect any particular cancer.

The doctor explains, however, that each possible therapy has its own risks and side-effects. The patient now has the information needed to make a decision on which treatment or combinations of treatments to choose. The person may require further information and advice from the doctor, or may even seek a second opinion from another specialist.

Ultimately, though, the patient has to make the decision based on what he or she considers most suitable. In this instance, chemotherapy may offer a better chance of success. Still, the patient may not want to endure the unpleasant side-effects of such treatment. So, the choice may be to have surgery with its attendant risks in order to gain its potential benefits.

Dr Geoffrey Riley and Professor Ralph Simmonds wrote on the subject in *The Medical Journal of Australia*: "It takes little thought to see that respect for the patient's autonomy is the preferred way to practice medicine. A patient's decisions will be made with many considerations beyond the purely medical ones being taken into account."

The reality is that today more and more people are deciding against blood transfusion and seeking alternatives. In a 1996 Canadian Gallup Poll, 89% of respondents said they would prefer an alternative if told they required blood transfusion for an operation. A survey conducted in Western Australia in 1998 found that 96% of those surveyed preferred an alternative to blood transfusion.

With the benefit of hindsight, one could ask: Had the alternatives to transfusion, developed in the late '50s and early '60s before the HIV era, been offered more widely to patients, how many lives might have been saved and how many tragedies avoided?

More importantly, one should now ask: Will the lessons of the past be learned? Proven and effective techniques and methods are available to avoid or minimize exposure to blood transfusion and, accordingly, potential tragedies in the future. Their application, however, requires a fundamental change from traditional practices.

Let us now look at what is involved in bloodless surgery and how it is done.

1   Estioko, Dr Manuel R., cardiovascular and thoracic surgeon with the Kay Medical Group for Cardiac, Vascular & Pulmonary Surgery; Medical Director of the Transfusion-Free Medicine and Surgery Center, Good Samaritan Hospital (GSH), Los Angeles, California, USA.

2   Spence, Dr Richard K., Director of Surgical Education for the Baptist Health Systems Hospitals, Alabama; Director, Alabama Center for Transfusion Alternatives.

3   Shander, Dr Aryeh, Assistant Professor of Anesthesiology, Mount Sinai School of Medicine, New York; Chief of the Department of Anesthesia, Critical Care, Hyperbaric Medicine, and the Center for Pain Control, Englewood Hospital; and Director of the New Jersey Institute for the Advancement of Bloodless Medicine and Surgery.

4   Spahn, Professor Donat, Professor of Anesthesiology, The Institute of Anesthesiology, University Hospital, Zurich, Switzerland.

5   Rosengart, Dr Todd, Associate Professor of Cardiothoracic Surgery, The New York Hospital – Cornell Medical Center, New York, NY.

6   Multimodality refers to the combined application of many methods and therapeutic agents. It is the key to "bloodless" management, as the reader will see in the next two chapters.

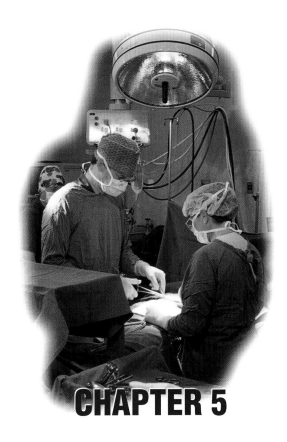

CHAPTER 5

BLOODLESS SURGERY - HOW IT WORKS

Chapter

Three Fundamental Aims

*B*loodless surgery demands a totally integrated team approach. The skills of surgeons, anesthesiologists, hematologists, pathologists and, indeed, all other specialists and support staff, combine to produce a whole new aspect of patient care.

In this exciting field of medical endeavor, the latest developments in technology fuse with the dedicated research of visionaries who seek a better way.

Though the tasks undertaken by bloodless surgery teams sound complex, the fundamental aims of their work can be expressed quite simply. These are to:

- Minimize blood loss;
- Maximize oxygen delivery;
- Maximize the body's ability to produce blood or, put another way, assist the body to becoming its own blood bank.

A patient choosing to undergo bloodless surgery soon realizes the program has three distinct, integrated stages. Moreover, he or she will discover the preparation before the operation (*preoperative phase*) and the treatment immediately after the procedure (*postoperative phase*) are regarded as being equally as important as the time spent on the operating table itself (*intraoperative phase*). The medical term encompassing all three stages from start to finish is *perioperative*.

The preoperative stage assesses and prepares patients, ensuring they are in the best possible condition for the operation. The postoperative phase requires specialists to minimize further blood loss and/or manage anemia that may have arisen from blood loss during surgery.

In emergencies or trauma, when there is little time for preparation, aggressive application of the intraoperative and postoperative phases is adopted.

While the surgeon and anesthesiologist have major roles, the success of what they do also depends on the vital contribution of hematologists, intensivists, pathologists, pharmacists and other appropriate specialists. Equally important to the team effort is the understanding and expertise of the various operating room, recovery room, ward, laboratory and hospital staff. This goes right through from the kitchen staff, where special diets may be required, to the office, admission and executive administration. Everyone involved in bloodless surgery understands its special pre-requisites and its all-important teamwork nature. Its success lies in this total approach.[1]

(1) The Preoperative Phase:

Assessment and Preparation

Bloodless surgery for an elective procedure begins long before the patient enters the operating room. An essential aspect is the preoperative assessment and work-up, designed to make sure the patient is in the best possible condition before the operation.

This stage essentially optimizes the patient's fitness for the operation and, more often than not, is handled by the anesthesiologist. For more complex operations or major surgery where hematological deficiencies or underlying diseases are identified, the surgeon or anesthesiologist normally refers the patient to a hematologist. On occasion, an intensive care or specialist physician is consulted for more comprehensive review and treatment. Where possible, all this takes place at least four weeks before surgery. Appraisals of this scope are seldom undertaken in medical practices or hospitals unfamiliar with bloodless surgery.

In the preoperative phase, the patient will be asked to provide a thorough medical history as well as submit to a general physical examination. The purpose here is to identify the limits of physiological reserves, optimize them and tailor the procedure to the individual's clinical circumstances.

At this early stage, it is also possible to identify and address factors which may contribute to extra bleeding during the operation:

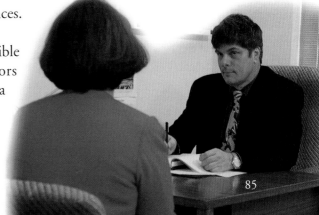

- A bleeding history will be conducted. Details of abnormal bleeding during childhood, previous surgery, dental extractions, pregnancy or abnormal nosebleeds or gum bleeding, abnormal bruising and so on can help establish if there are any coagulation problems.

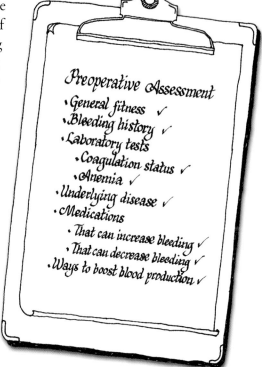

Preoperative Assessment
- General fitness ✓
- Bleeding history ✓
- Laboratory tests
  - Coagulation status ✓
  - Anemia ✓
- Underlying disease ✓
- Medications
  - That can increase bleeding ✓
  - That can decrease bleeding ✓
- Ways to boost blood production ✓

- Laboratory tests can then identify specific defects in the clotting process, such as deficiency in one of the blood clotting factors, low platelet numbers or platelet dysfunction (remember, platelets are an important element in coagulation). Sometimes these signify underlying disease, such as liver or kidney disorder, which may require treatment before surgery.

- Several medications can contribute to bleeding during an operation. Aspirin, for example, interferes with platelet function. Some analgesic and anti-inflammatory drugs can interfere with coagulation. Similarly, high-dose antibiotic therapy and some diuretics can hinder the body's blood-clotting ability. If the patient is on any of these medications, an appropriate specialist will consider how best to approach this, possibly changing or stopping the medication well before the operation.

As well as eliminating factors that can increase bleeding, in this preoperative stage doctors can also consider the options offered to them by a range of specially designed medications known as hemostatic agents. These can be given before, during or after the surgery to help reinforce the coagulation system and further reduce bleeding.

Boosting the Blood Factory

Doctors will check hemoglobin levels and the patient's ability to make blood. Anemia can be caused by disease, deficiencies or even chronic bleeding from the condition the surgery is planned to treat. As part of preoperative preparations, hematologists will look at ways of building hemoglobin back to near-normal, normal, or, even above-normal levels.

It may be necessary to replenish or supplement the building blocks for blood cell formation. The body's ability to make blood depends on the presence of a range of essential ingredients. Among these are iron, vitamins, amino acids and hormones. Equally important is a person's ability to absorb and synthesize these essential ingredients. Should any of them be absent or depleted, blood manufacture is impaired.

Meanwhile, there are specialized medications that can boost the body's blood-making ability more rapidly. One of these is synthetically produced *erythropoietin*, commonly referred to by its abbreviation — EPO. This is a naturally occurring hormone that stimulates the body's red blood cell production. When the kidneys detect that more red blood cells are needed, they release natural erythropoietin which, in turn, travels via the blood stream around to the bone marrow. There the additional cells are manufactured.

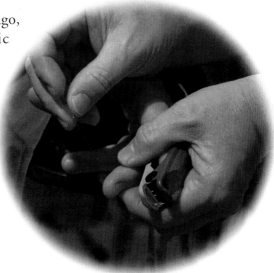

A little more than a decade ago, scientists applied genetic engineering technology to produce EPO in the laboratory (recombinant human erythropoietin — *epoetin alfa*).[2] When this synthetically produced substance is injected into an anemic patient[3], the body quickly manufactures new red blood cells.

Administered at the appropriate time before an operation, EPO helps to correct anemia and, at the same time, ensures the body is fully primed and ready to replace blood lost during surgery. The benefits for the recovery period, thus incurred, are obvious. Preoperative use of EPO alone can significantly reduce the amount of donor blood required.

Using Your Own Blood

A brochure published by the American Red Cross once advised: "Your own blood (autologous blood) is the safest blood available because it is always compatible and eliminates any possibility of transfusion-related problems."

Several autologous blood options are available. One is to have your own blood collected and stored before your operation, referred to as *preoperative autologous blood donation* (PABD). This usually starts about three to four weeks before your operation. Sometimes, supplements and medications such as EPO are given to stimulate blood production, enabling you to have more blood collected and stored.

While predonating one's own blood for subsequent autologous transfusion is a means of avoiding blood from another person, there are some limitations. For instance, patients in poor health, or with serious heart disease may not be able to donate their own blood safely.

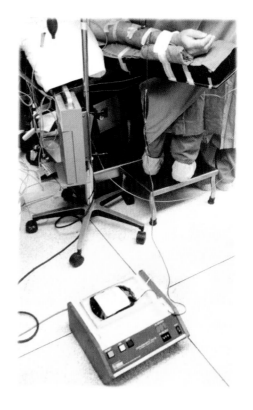

Predonated blood has to be stored and is therefore subject to the same deterioration as other stored blood. This means predonated blood, like the allogeneic variety, may have a decreased ability to release oxygen and be subject to the same complications from breakdown products. Like other stored blood, predonated blood quickly loses its clotting factors. In addition, there is the risk of bacterial contamination. Some patients have experienced serious reactions to their own stored blood.

One body of professional opinion argues that predonating blood lacks cost-effectiveness. Like all donated blood, predonated autologous blood still has to be screened, tested and properly identified to avoid possible mix-up and all this involves considerable expense. More recent expert opinion suggests a broader calculation must be made. Into the equation must be factored the expense of short-term and long-term complications of allogeneic blood and their treatment. Predonated autologous blood then becomes very cost-effective.

An article in the British publication, *ABC of Transfusion* (1998) supported autologous transfusions from a different viewpoint. The main benefit of autologous blood, the article noted, was likely to be avoidance of an unknown risk. It went on: "For instance, there may be an infectious agent of long incubation spreading in the population, which might be transmissible by transfusion and for which no screening test is yet available. In the UK, the most obvious potential threat at present is variant Creutzfeldt-Jakob disease (CJD), but experiences with HIV and hepatitis C indicate that we must not be complacent about as yet unrecognized viruses."

And so, while not acceptable to those with religious objections to blood, the reader should appreciate that predonated blood is another avenue open to those who choose to avoid donor blood. It does have distinct advantages and, apart from clerical error, it most certainly removes the risks of contracting infectious disease from someone else's blood. In operations where blood may become a consideration, two units collected just two weeks before surgery should cover most situations and minimize the time in storage.

Other autologous blood transfusion options are available known as *hemodilution, component sequestration* and various forms of what is generally referred to as intra- and postoperative *cell salvage*. These are discussed in Chapter 6.

(2) The Intraoperative Phase:

Surgical Techniques

The first two principles of bloodless surgery apply prominently in stage two when the operation is performed — minimizing blood loss and maximizing oxygen delivery. The surgeon will adopt meticulous surgical techniques, initially making the smallest possible incision and then, as he or she continues, quickly stopping all bleeding no matter how minor. This is the cornerstone of bloodless surgery. Skill, experience and the ability to proceed expeditiously are keys to minimizing blood loss.

In the past, it was common to cut right through to the "work site." Avoiding blood loss was not considered to be a major priority since it could always be replaced by a standby supply of banked blood. Consequently, there was considerable blood loss and the need for replacement by transfusion.

With the "bloodless" approach, the emphasis is on smaller incisions together with careful and gentle working through less vascular layers of tissue, stopping all the bleeding on the way. Smaller vessels are sealed with surgical devices designed to cut and coagulate simultaneously. Larger vessels are either cauterized before being cut or sometimes clamped or tied off. This is what's called *meticulous hemostasis*, meticulous attention to stopping all bleeding. This surgical approach alone plays a major role in reducing bleeding and, subsequently, blood transfusion.

The 1995 Consensus Conference on blood management said of meticulous hemostasis: "Its impact on the transfusion decision is clear: blood that is not lost does not have to be replaced." It combines the use of clever new instruments and products with a revised approach aimed at minimizing the amount of bleeding during surgery.[4] Again, more details are given in Chapter 6.

Other techniques involve temporarily isolating the blood supply to very vascular organs, such as the liver, with clips, clamps and similar devices before surgery begins. The blood supply can then be restored when the operation is finished.

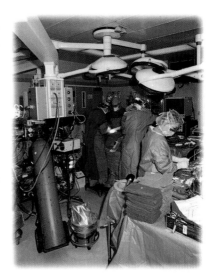

Certain medications injected locally into the operation's target area are sometimes used to constrict or "shrink" the blood vessels and thereby decrease blood flow to that area.

In some procedures on the extremities, for example, knee replacement, a pneumatic tourniquet can be applied above the surgical site, producing a bloodless field in which to operate.

Bleeding can often be reduced during surgery by positioning the patient on the table so that the operation site is above the level of the heart. Additionally, care must be taken to avoid any pressure on major veins which can increase bleeding.

Another technique is *arterial embolization*. Here a catheter is inserted into an artery to introduce a balloon or some other material, thereby closing off the vessels feeding the surgical area. This can be done before, during or after the operation and has proven very effective in surgery on

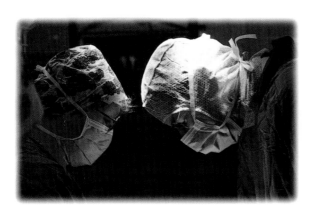

brain and bone tumors or fractures of the pelvis. The method has also been used in emergencies to arrest hemorrhage in the pelvic and abdominal areas.

"The surgeon should enter the operating room with the goal of preventing as much blood loss as possible by maintaining careful surgical hemostasis."

Richard Spence MD
Emerging Trends in Surgical Blood Transfusion. *Seminars in Hematology* 1997;34(3):48-53.

"Blood loss is an inevitable consequence of surgery. However, large differences in the amount of perioperative blood loss between surgeons and institutions lead to the conclusion that there is limited awareness of the risks of anaemia and that strategies to reduce blood loss are not used frequently."

H. Gombotz, MD, et al.
Methods for reduction of perioperative bleeding. *Br J Anaesth.* 1998;81(Suppl 1):62-66.

Saving Time, Saving Blood

Not surprisingly, the time taken to complete an operation has direct bearing on the amount of blood lost. This highlights the importance of teamwork in the operating room. The operating room staff need to have a thorough understanding of the surgeon's techniques and preferences. They must anticipate his needs and timing and have everything ready when required.

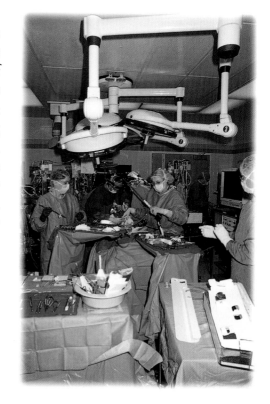

Addressing the Paris 1996 bloodless surgery conference, orthopedic surgeon, Richard Coombs, defined the most important factor in reducing the requirement for blood transfusion as "very careful preoperative planning." He said: "With such preparation, it has been possible to reduce the time taken, even for a hip revision procedure[5] to 50 minutes or less in selected cases." To help ensure this expeditious surgery, every piece of equipment is made immediately available when needed.

In certain complex operations, more than one surgeon may be involved, further reducing operating time and blood loss. Some difficult procedures can even be done in stages, allowing for hemoglobin recovery between operations.

Anesthetic techniques

The anesthesiologist works very closely with the surgeon to minimize blood loss and plays the key role in maintaining oxygen delivery to the cells. Attention to the choice of anesthetic agent and technique, fluid and oxygen administration, mode of ventilation, medications, muscle relaxants, control of blood pressure and body temperature, positioning of the patient on the operating table, blood collection and recycling techniques and pain control are all vital elements. You will find expanded references to these in the next chapter.

Hypotensive Anesthesia

One option is known as *hypotensive anesthesia* or *controlled deliberate hypotension*, by which the patient's blood pressure is lowered, using either medications or anesthetic techniques. Blood is pumped under pressure through the vessels around the body and, as with a damaged garden hose, when the tap is turned down the volume of escaping fluid decreases. A similar principle applies with controlled hypotension and this technique alone can reduce blood loss in certain procedures by as much as 70% and operating time by up to 30%.

The Use of Non-blood Fluids

During surgery, the anesthesiologist has available a variety of non-blood fluids which may be administered to maintain a patient's blood volume.

They are known as *volume expanders*. The body can compensate and cope with considerable blood loss as long as fluid volume is replaced, thus maintaining blood pressure and circulation to the organs. Some of these fluids, such as normal saline and Ringer's solution provide immediate volume expansion but do not stay in the vascular system for long. Remember, normal saline solution had limitations during World War II in treating massive hemorrhage because it did not remain in the vascular system long enough. Conversely, some of the synthetic colloid expanders such as *pentastarch*, *hetastarch*, *dextran* and *gelatin* preparations are specifically designed to stay in the vascular system for longer periods.

We described earlier how the loss of large amounts of blood can deplete plasma proteins such as albumin. This sometimes causes fluid to leak into the tissue, in turn, bringing on pulmonary edema and compromizing oxygen delivery. One way to address this problem is to administer human albumin derived from donated plasma. However, an alternative is to use synthetic colloid volume expanders designed to work like albumin. When administered, these increase the osmotic pressure and are able to pull the fluid in the tissue back into the veins.

Non-blood fluids are also used for deliberately diluting a patient's blood — a blood conservation technique known as hemodilution, which is described more fully later.

A number of other techniques may be used intraoperatively, including hypothermia, hyperoxic ventilation, salvaging and recycling blood and the use of medications that reduce bleeding. These and others are also discussed in Chapter 6.

As with most things, practice makes perfect. So it is with bloodless surgery. Its success depends on an experienced team practiced at putting together all these techniques.

(3) The Postoperative Phase:

In all surgery, the postoperative phase requires very careful monitoring of all patients; to awaken them from anesthesia and stabilize them ready to return to the ward.

Minimizing Blood Loss

In addition to the usual postoperative patient monitoring, careful attention is given to reduce further blood loss, maximize blood production and support oxygen needs. With some operations, there can be as much bleeding after the procedure as during it. For example, with orthopedic surgery, bones which have been cut during the operation may continue to ooze for up to 24 hours or more afterwards. With knee replacement surgery, often carried out with a tourniquet above the knee, most blood loss happens after the operation.

At the end of an operation, drains are inserted into the wound. Through a tube, the blood is collected in a bottle — a common sight alongside a patient's bed after an operation. After surgery, where there may be considerable postoperative blood loss, what is known as a cell salvage machine can be attached to the drains to collect the blood. The machine washes the blood, then returns it to the patient. This is known as postoperative blood salvage.

Pharmacological agents, such as *desmopressin*, can also be administered to reduce and control postoperative bleeding. (See Appendix 2 p. 153).

It is important to distinguish between normal postoperative blood loss, such as that from an oozing wound, and the more severe circumstance in which bleeding may have resulted from a loose suture, or even a vessel that has

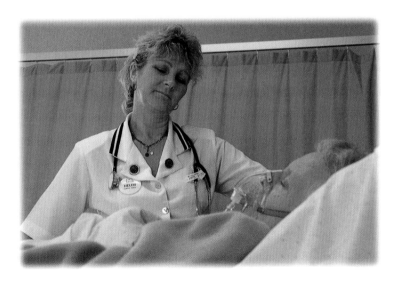

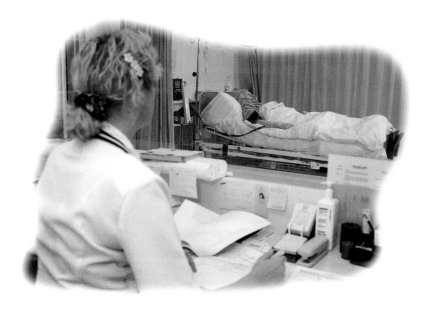

been cut and not identified. Such bleeding almost certainly will require prompt reoperation. With patients who refuse blood under any circumstance, immediate control of active bleeding is vital. Any delay could place them in jeopardy.

Minimizing Blood Sampling

As part of the careful monitoring of patients in the postoperative stage, blood samples need to be taken for analysis. If careful attention is not given to the amount removed and to the number of samples taken, a patient can unnecessarily lose a lot of blood to the apparent demands of the laboratory. This is clinically referred to as *iatrogenic* (doctor-induced) anemia. Studies have shown that patients can lose up to 1.3 liters this way during their hospital stay. Extraordinary as it may seem, a transfusion is sometimes given to replace blood removed for testing. Such a situation can pose particularly serious problems for small children and babies who have only small blood volumes.

Microsampling techniques significantly reduce the quantity of blood taken for this purpose. Using microsampling, most tests can be performed with less than one milliliter of blood. This compares with normal sampling's range varying from 4 mls to 20 mls per tube, per test.

Maximizing Blood Production After an Operation

A number of medications are available to speed the body's ability to replace significant or unexpected blood-loss during an operation. These complement the careful preoperative phase in elective surgery, or are used more aggressively at this point in emergency surgery or trauma where there is insufficient time to prepare the patient.

Among these medications, iron, understandably, is very important. Iron taken orally will be sufficient in some situations, but this has its limitations. After surgery, the patient's ability to absorb iron is often compromised or there is a need to replenish quickly iron stores for rapid red cell production. Intravenous administration is a more effective way to replace acutely lost iron. This is despite the historic fears of many doctors whose reluctance to use intravenous iron is based on severe allergic reactions experienced by some patients in years past. Newer preparations and improved methods of administration have virtually eliminated such complications today.

Along with special attention to nutrition, sometimes administered intravenously, other vitamins and blood-building medications may be given, not least of all EPO.

If EPO is used at this juncture, higher than normal doses may be required to speed up production. It is rather like pushing your foot harder on the accelerator to make your car go faster. If the accelerator is pressed down hard, there also needs to be fuel in the tank for the car to react accordingly. It is essential all the fuel or support medication for red cell production — iron, folic acid, vitamin B 12 — also be given, or EPO won't work effectively.

Consider this situation: many doctors inexperienced in EPO's use object initially to administering it. They maintain it takes too long to work. But, as it often happens, two or three days later they still have an anemic patient who has not been given EPO. By this time it could have been working. Although there is a lag period, in appropriate EPO doses, *reticulocytes* (immature red blood cells) are released from the bone marrow within minutes to hours. New mature red blood cells are produced within one to three days. Beneficial rises in hemoglobin levels have been seen within the first week.

Therefore, the use of EPO can play an important role in restoring lost blood at the postoperative stage of bloodless surgery. At the same time, while EPO specifically stimulates the production of red blood cells, some investigators have also seen an occasional slight rise in platelet production.

Stimulating Blood Cell Production

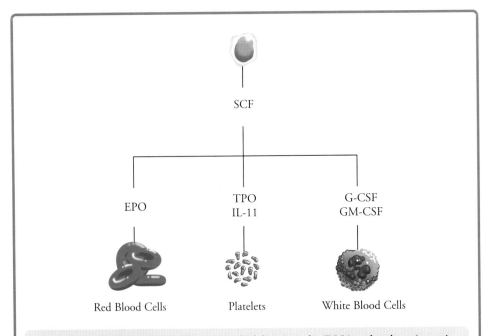

EPO	TPO IL-11	G-CSF GM-CSF
Red Blood Cells	Platelets	White Blood Cells

Synthetic medications manufactured in the laboratory by DNA technology (genetic engineering) stimulate blood cell production. These are referred to as recombinant hematopoietic growth factors. When administered they replicate the body's natural stimulating factors and "rev up" the production of specific blood cells. For example, erythropoietin (EPO) specifically drives the production of red blood cells, Colony Stimulating Factors (GM-CSF, G-CSF) drive the production of certain white blood cells and newer products such as Interleukin-11 (IL-11) and Thrombopoietin (TPO) have been developed to stimulate platelet production. A number of other innovations, including Stem Cell Factor (SCF) which stimulates the production of stem cells, are presently undergoing clinical trials.

The Transfusion Trigger in Perspective

It is important to understand that lower and, sometimes, much lower hemoglobin levels may be acceptable. For many years the decision to give a blood transfusion (the "transfusion trigger") was based on a set "blood count" or hemoglobin level of 10 g/dL. When it fell to 10 g/dL from the normal average of 16 g/dL for men, or 14 g/dL for women, a blood transfusion was considered essential. As explained in the last chapter, this guideline had little scientific basis, but became the accepted creed in all medical textbooks. The "10/30 rule" as it was called (a hemoglobin of 10 g/dL or a hematocrit of 30%), was applied equally to men and women, despite the disparity in their normal hemoglobin levels.

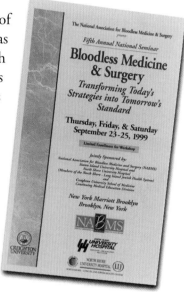

The practice, however, has failed to stand the test of critical examination during the past decade. It has become apparent that most patients can tolerate much lower hemoglobin levels as long as normal volume is maintained. The 1988 NIH Transfusion Consensus Conference, referred to earlier, suggested the transfusion level be lowered to 7 g/dL in patients without heart disease, or those who showed no symptoms of suffering from a lower hemoglobin level.

In 1996 and 1998, respectively, the American Society of Anesthesiologists and the College of American Pathologists published practice guidelines in which they stated hemoglobins as low as 6 g/dL might be acceptable in certain patients showing no symptoms of anemia. Both stressed that the decision to transfuse should not be based on a single hemoglobin figure, but rather on clinical indicators for each patient's needs. Professor Edwin Deitch[6], speaking at a conference in 1999[7], said experience suggested hemoglobins as low as 5-6 g/dL might be acceptable in patients without heart disease. Patients with heart disease, such as narrowing of the coronary arteries, appear to be less able to compensate for anemia and possibly are at increased risk. These patients may require more aggressive management.

Much has been learned from those who rejected transfusions for religious reasons and whose subsequent treatment demonstrated they could survive on extremely low blood counts — as low, indeed, as 1.4 g/dL. At the 1999 New York conference[8], Dr Aryeh Shander explained how 24 such patients at his hospital, all with acute, massive blood loss, had been successfully managed with blood levels below 5 g/dL. One patient had a hemoglobin level of 1.7 g/dL, five had 2 g/dL, eight had 3 g/dL and ten less than 5 g/dL.

The patients required special, aggressive management without the use of blood. While hemoglobin levels this low are not ideal and there are risks involved, it does demonstrate that with appropriate management these patients can survive.

A special issue of *Time* magazine in 1997, cited the case of 32-year-old, Henry Jackson, whose hemoglobin had dropped from 13 g/dL to 1.7 g/dL as a result of massive internal bleeding. The report described how Jackson, who refused a blood transfusion for religious reasons, was transferred unconscious from one hospital to the Englewood Hospital's New Jersey Institute for the Advancement of Bloodless Medicine and Surgery. At Englewood, Dr Shander's team moved quickly to reduce the patient's need for oxygen, using drugs to stem the demand by the muscles, brain, lungs and other organs. Jackson was also put on a ventilator

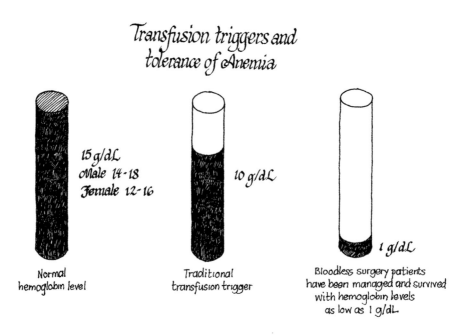

Transfusion triggers and
tolerance of Anemia

15 g/dL
Male 14-18
Female 12-16

Normal
hemoglobin level

10 g/dL

Traditional
transfusion trigger

1 g/dL

Bloodless surgery patients
have been managed and survived
with hemoglobin levels
as low as 1 g/dL

to supply extra oxygen and further reduce his body's workload. Next, the team administered large doses of iron and vitamin supplements, along with synthetic EPO to stimulate the production of red blood cells. Volume expanders were given to replace the fluid in the circulatory system which had been drastically depleted by the loss of almost 90% of his blood.

Time reported how Jackson recovered from that point. Within four days, his blood hemoglobin level had increased dramatically and, soon after, he was able to talk about his own remarkable recovery — much to his own amazement as well as that of the first hospital's official who called to ask whether the patient had died. Far from being dead, the patient was ready to be discharged and resume his normal life.

Many other documented medical experiences like this have undoubtedly helped contribute to the revision of the transfusion trigger. At the same time, they have helped reduce further the use of blood.

Indeed, the acceptance of a lower hemoglobin level has become a strategy in itself to avoid transfusion. Professor Terri Monk[9] (pictured left) told the 1999 New York conference: "One alternative to a blood transfusion is 'no transfusion or a lowering of the transfusion trigger.' Transfusion guidelines state there is no clear and specific hemoglobin level below which patients require transfusing."

Current thinking is that the decision to transfuse should not be based on a single hemoglobin or laboratory value. Rather, it should be determined by a patient's highly individualized needs. The patient's physiological indications must be taken into account as must his or her oxygen requirements.

"The age-old transfusion trigger of a hemoglobin level of 100 g/L (10 g/dL) is no longer defensible. Physiologic evidence and clinical experience point to a remarkable human tolerance of low hemoglobin levels. Healthy patients can withstand hemoglobin levels between 50 g/L and 70 g/L without adverse effects. The decision to

give a transfusion clearly depends on the clinical condition of an individual patient."

H. G. Welch, K. R. Meehan, L. T. Goodnough.
Prudent Strategies for Elective Red Blood Cell Transfusion.
Annals of Internal Medicine. 1992;116:393-402.

"The data preclude any scientific conclusions in support of a "safe" Hb [hemoglobin] concentration or transfusion trigger. However, clinicians may be reassured by the absence of mortality due to anemia in patients with hemoglobin concentrations between 5 and 7 g/dL...The possibility of survival with severe anemia...is supported by the experience of one author who stated that 73 patients with preoperative Hb concentrations less than 5 g/dL underwent surgery without subsequent mortality... Survival is possible at extremely low oxygen-carrying capacity – Hb concentrations as low as 1.4 g/dL – but that mortality (with an unknown incidence) is encountered at Hb concentrations less than 5 g/dL."

M. K. Viele, R. B. Weiskopf.
What can we learn about the need for transfusion from patients who refuse blood? *Transfusion* 1994;34(5):396-401.

PREOPERATIVE

Assessment & Work-up
Surgeon/ Anesthesiologist/ Intensivist/ Hematologist

- Assess patient's fitness for operation
- Hematological analysis
  - bleeding history
  - laboratory tests
  - anemia
  - coagulation status
- Correct underlying disorders
- Assess ways to reduce surgical bleeding
- Maximize hemopoiesis iron, EPO, folate, Vit B12, nutrition, Vit C and others.

INTRAOPERATIVE

Surgical/ Anesthetic/ Pharmacological strategies to minimize blood loss and maximize oxygen availability and delivery

- Meticulous surgical technique and hemostasis
- Arterial embolization
- Local vasoconstrictive agents
- Topical hemostats
- Tourniquet
- Reduced operating time
- Patient positioning
- Minimally invasive surgery
- Enlarged operative team
- Staging complex procedures
- Controlled hemodilution
- Hypotensive anesthesia/ Controlled deliberate hypotension
- Hypothermia (for specific situations, otherwise, maintain normothermia)
- Autologous cell salvage
- Autologous component sequestration
- Judicious use of fluids
- Appropriate oxygen support
- Pharmacological agents to reduce bleeding

POSTOPERATIVE

Intensivists/hematologists/hyperbaric physicians/other specialists

- Minimize blood loss
  - Monitor patient and promptly arrest postoperative bleeding
  - Microsampling
  - Postoperative blood salvage
  - Prompt reoperation to stop active bleeding
- Maximize blood production
  - EPO, iron, folate, B12, nutrition
- Maximize oxygen delivery
  - Maximize cardiac output
  - Maximize oxygen supply
  - Appropriate fluid administration
  - Hyperbaric oxygen therapy
- Minimize oxygen consumption
  - Reduce metabolic rate
  Sedation, paralysis, hypothermia

1   Many operations performed are minor procedures such as those for ingrown toe-nails, hernia repairs and so on. Blood transfusion would rarely, if ever, be a consideration for these. If in doubt, patients are advised to ask their doctor if the operation has the risk of significant blood loss and, therefore, a transfusion.

2   Some synthetic erythropoietin preparations have had human albumin, derived from plasma, added to the medication as a stabilizer.

3   The reader needs to be aware there are different types of anemia resulting from various causes. Some, for example, linked to bone marrow failure, may not respond to EPO treatment.

4   This approach is in fact not new. American pioneer surgeon, William Halsted (1852-1922) who established the first surgical school in the US at Johns Hopkins University, Baltimore, emphasized gentle handling of tissue, attention to detail and meticulous hemostasis. Concern over the safety of blood has seen a re-emphasis of his principles. As Dr Richard Spence wrote in the journal *Seminars in Hematology*, "Surgeons are relearning Halstedian principles of gentle tissue handling, anatomic dissection, and blood loss minimization in all operations."

5   A re-operation to remove and replace an artificial hip – a more complex and bloody operation than the original hip procedure.

6   Deitch, Dr Edwin, Professor and Chairman, Department of Surgery, New Jersey Medical School, Newark, New Jersey. In Hong Kong he was speaking on the subject, "Practices and Physiology of Bloodless Therapy in Emergency Surgery and the ICU."

7   At Asia's first International Bloodless Medicine and Surgery Conference in Hong Kong (Aug 1999).

8   Bloodless Medicine and Surgery: Transforming Today's Strategies into Tomorrow's Standard.(Sept 1999)

9   Monk, Professor Terri, Professor, Department of Anesthesiology, University of Florida, Gainesville, Florida. She spoke at the conference on the subject "The Role of the Anesthesiologist in a Bloodless Medicine and Surgery Program."

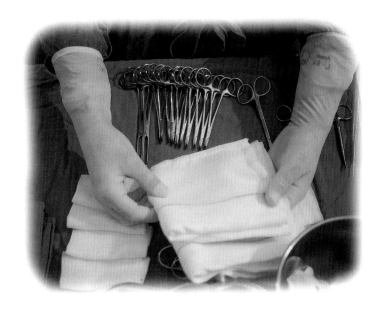

CHAPTER 6

BLOODLESS SURGERY'S "TOOLBOX"

- *Iron Therapy: Why it is so Important*
- *Instruments and Pharmacological Products*
- *Medications that Help Coagulation*
- *"Keyhole" Surgery*
- *What is Hemodilution?*
- *Hypothermia*
- *Salvaging and Recycling*
- *Oxygen Support*
- *Helping the Body to Compensate*
- *Hyperbaric Oxygen Therapy*
- *Management of Trauma*

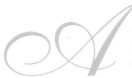s with any highly skilled profession, the craftsmen of bloodless surgery rely heavily on their specialized "toolbox."

Some of the medications, methods and equipment to be found there have, in fact, been around a long time. What makes the difference is how the "old gear" is now employed and this all really comes down to the bloodless craftsmen's finely tuned surgical art. But, of course, there is that section of the "toolbox" where the very latest in technological progress is continually expanding the contents.

Here can be found sophisticated tools with names like argon beam coagulators, ultrasonic scalpels, water-jet dissectors, automated cell salvage machines, laparoscopes and such like. This is also where you'll find a specialist range of strange-sounding medications and substances. There are recombinant blood producing and clotting factors and new generation synthetic volume expanders. There are oxygen therapeutics and gene therapy and hemostatic agents which cover a multitude of drugs, staples, tacks, meshes, pastes, sponges, pads, powders and biological glues.[1]

In this chapter we examine more closely the ever-expanding bloodless surgery toolbox.

Iron Therapy: Why it is so Important

Iron is an essential ingredient in blood production. The hemoglobin in red blood cells is made up partly of iron, each hemoglobin molecule containing four iron atoms to which oxygen binds for transport. The bulk of the body's iron (65-75%) is present in our hemoglobin, with the remainder held as storage, mostly in the bone marrow. To manufacture hemoglobin, the body uses iron from storage and recycles iron from worn-out red blood cells.

An average adult male needs approximately 1 mg of iron a day for hemoglobin production and storage. An average adult female, however, needs 2 mg to compensate for blood lost through menstruation. Likewise, a pregnant woman will absorb up to 3 mg of her daily intake to provide for her own needs and that of the fetus. A child needs around 2 mg to allow for normal daily blood production and meet the additional demands essential for growth.

If supply does not keep up with demand, the body is not able to produce a normal quantity of healthy red blood cells and a person may develop what is known as iron deficiency anemia — the most common form of human anemia. There is a delicate balance between the amount of iron we absorb and lose on a daily basis. Although the average western diet provides an intake of 15 - 20 mg a day, we absorb only some 10% of that, or about 1-1.5 mg and lose an almost equal amount daily in the feces and sweat. With such a tenuous balance, iron stores can be depleted by inadequate diet, poor absorption or, most commonly, from chronic or acute blood loss. Each milliliter of blood contains approximately 0.5 mg of iron and, so, losing blood means losing iron. Depleted iron stores may need to be replaced, once the cause and type of anemia have been identified. There are other forms of anemia that simply do not respond to iron therapy alone.

A good diet of iron-rich foods can help maintain and replenish iron levels, along with foods containing vitamin C which helps the absorption process. Interestingly, in iron deficiency anemia, the body is able to increase its absorption of iron to about 25% of the iron ingested.

Most meat and fish dishes provide an excellent source of iron, supported by a select range of greens, dried fruit, beans, grains and iron fortified cereals. These two groups of food are also strong sources of vitamin B_{12} and folic acid, both necessary to assist with the formation of red blood cells.

Treatment of iron deficiency anemia may include iron supplements. Oral iron is usually the preferred and easiest means of iron administration. However, its effect will be determined by the type of preparation, appropriate dose and the body's ability to absorb it.

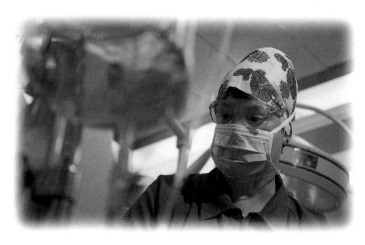

Iron is most readily absorbed in the upper part of the small intestine, primarily the duodenum. Slow release or enteric-coated iron tablets take iron past these high absorption sites to the lower intestine where it is poorly absorbed. Some liquid iron preparations and non-coated tablets that release iron in the upper intestine provide better absorption. Taking ascorbic acid (vitamin C) can also increase absorption.

It is important to note that some foods and medications can decrease iron absorption if taken at the same time as iron supplements. It has been recommended that iron supplements be taken one hour before or two hours after milk, tea, coffee and eggs. A separate table here lists these drug and food interactions.

Sometimes, it may be necessary to administer iron intravenously to replace that depleted during acute blood loss. Intravenous administration may also be necessary to sustain the large amounts of iron required to keep pace with the stimulation of erythropoietin treatment. In all circumstances, intravenous iron needs to be administered in a hospital by an experienced doctor.

All treatments associated with iron therapy should be performed in consultation with your doctor.

DRUG AND FOOD INTERACTIONS

Concurrent use with the following products can decrease iron absorption. Take iron supplements one hour before or two hours after these preparations: -

- Milk or milk products
- Eggs
- Coffee
- Tea (contains tannic acid)
- Whole-grain breads and cereals (contain phytic acid)
- Dietary fibre
- Antacids containing carbonates or magnesium trisilicate
- Calcium supplements
- Histamine H_2 – receptor antagonists (such as cimetidine)
- Omeprazole
- Pancreatin or pancrelipase

A Word of Caution

Patients on the following medications should be aware that iron may decrease the absorption of their drug intake. Medications should not be taken within two hours of taking iron supplements.

- Tetracyclines
- Quinolones (ciprofloxacin)
- Penicillamine
- Levodopa
- Methyldopa
- Etidronate

Note: Iron supplements, like all medications, should be kept out of reach of children. Iron tablet poisoning is one of the most common causes of infant poisoning.

Instruments and Pharmacological Products

In addition to the surgical techniques discussed in Chapter 5, the surgeon has valuable equipment at his disposal to achieve the overall goal of reducing blood loss. One of these is *electrocautery*, basically a hot wire or blade which uses heat generated by electrical energy either to seal off or simultaneously cut and coagulate bleeding vessels.

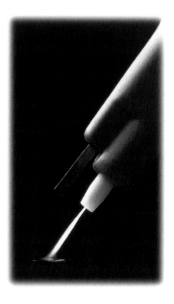

Ultrasonic scalpels accomplish much the same end using a different method. Ultrasonic energy vibrates the blade at up to 55,500 cycles a second, producing a characteristic humming sound, cutting and coagulating at the same time. This method generates a much lower temperature than electrocautery, causing less tissue damage.

Another device is the *argon beam coagulator* (pictured right). This works on a different principle to achieve a similar objective. Looking a bit like a miniature high-tech flame-thrower, it directs a stream of argon gas that blows the blood away from the surface, simultaneously acting as a conductor for radio frequency energy, which cauterizes the site. The surgeon uses the argon beam coagulator much like an airbrush, stroking it over the bleeding surface which brings about almost immediate hemostasis. This method of coagulation also does less tissue damage and further reduces tissue handling. There are numerous other devices like these, such as *lasers, microwave scalpels* and *water jet dissectors*. They accomplish the same purpose and are suited to particular types of surgical procedures. (See list in Appendix 2.)

Additional aids to reduce and control blood loss are a range of products known as *topical hemostatic agents*. These include packs, pads, sponges, pastes, powders, meshes, solutions and special dressings which, when applied to the wound — either tissue or bone — help promote clotting. Certain biological glues made from components of the patient's own blood such as fibrin, thrombin and platelets, may also be used to seal off bleeding surfaces.

Medications that Help Coagulation

There are special medications which, when injected or infused, further help reduce blood loss during an operation. Among these is *aprotinin*, which appears to have a two-fold action.

Firstly, it is believed to act as a protector of platelets which otherwise can be damaged. They can lose their blood-clotting viability as they bounce around in the tubing of either a heart-lung machine or cell salvage machine. Similarly, aprotinin is believed to overcome the problems of platelet damage from aspirin and antibiotics.

Secondly, it appears aprotinin also has an effect on the blood clotting process. It is what doctors call an *antifibrinolytic* and enables a stronger clot to be formed before being broken down. Medical reports suggest that the use of aprotinin can reduce blood loss in first-time heart surgery by up to 50% and, in repeat heart surgery, by as much as 80%. Used in orthopedic surgery, a decrease in blood loss of 26% has been reported. Surgeons have also achieved encouraging reductions in blood loss during liver transplants and in obstetric and gynecological procedures.

Note: A list of other hemostatic medications that act on facets of the coagulation system and reduce bleeding is on page 154.

"Keyhole" Surgery

Minimally invasive surgery (such as laparoscopic and endoscopic procedures), where surgeons operate using specialized instruments inserted in the patient through small incisions, is a very advanced and sophisticated technique. This way, doctors seek to minimize both blood loss and patient trauma. Otherwise known as *"keyhole surgery"*, it avoids the need for large incisions and allows the surgeon to proceed via a tiny camera. Also inserted in the body, the camera projects a television image of the operation site and the instruments in use. Such operations are, in essence, a remote control approach and very effective for certain conditions. Generally, recovery is faster and patients are out of hospital much sooner than those undergoing conventional open operations. Even complex heart procedures are now being performed this way.

However, with some patients who have anatomical abnormalities, or scarring from previous surgery, the risk of blood loss may be even higher with minimally invasive surgery. The very nature of the technique restricts the surgeon's view of the operation site. It therefore poses the risk of the surgeon failing to spot bleeding that is taking place out of camera view. Even when the bleeding site is identified, the functioning of the laparoscopic instruments is such that it takes a little time to stop it. Minimally invasive techniques are clearly not always the complete answer. [2]

Understanding Fluid Administration

Some 60% of the body's weight is water. This varies according to age, sex and build. Body water is contained in what are referred to as compartments (the interior of cells, the interior of blood vessels, or the space between cells). Intracellular fluid (water inside cells) constitutes two thirds of total body water. The other third is extracellular fluid (water outside the cells). The extracellular fluid is contained within two major compartments, the vascular or intravascular space (water within the blood vessels — in the plasma), making up about 25%, and the interstitial space (water outside the blood vessels and surrounding the cells), containing the remaining 75% of extracellular fluid. These compartments are divided by permeable membranes (the blood vessels' walls and the cells' membranes). Water moves through the membranes to these various compartments and its distribution depends on the substances dissolved or suspended in it and the permeability of the membranes. The body requires the volume of water in each of these compartments to be in the right balance for good health.

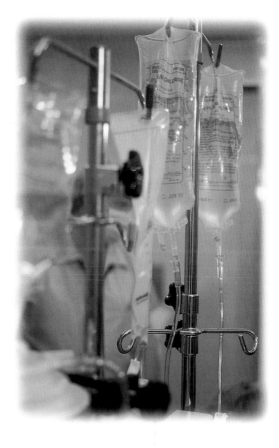

Volume expanders are designed essentially to replace loss of body water as a result of bleeding. They come in a variety of formulations to meet clinical needs. Their ingredients and formulation will determine to which compartment or compartments they will go and in what proportion, how quickly they will get there and for how long they will stay.

There are two groups of volume expanders, *crystalloids* and *colloids*. Crystalloids are solutions of water with salts (electrolytes) and/or sugars dissolved in them. They include normal saline, Ringer's solution and dextrose, to name a few. Colloids contain small particles of proteins, or other material such as starch or gelatin, mixed but not dissolved in water. Included in this group are pentastarch, hetastarch, dextran and gelatin. Serum albumin, derived from human plasma, is also used as a colloid volume expander.

Because of their make-up, when most crystalloid volume expanders are injected, they distribute both to the interstitial and vascular space. With some of these, 75% goes to the interstitial and 25% to the vascular space. In order to maintain intravascular blood volume with a crystalloid, clearly four times the amount of fluid needs to be given. Within hours, most of this fluid is removed from the body, mainly in the urine. Crystalloids are often the volume expander of choice. They provide immediate temporary volume expansion, are inexpensive, and considered to be safe, non-toxic and reaction-free. They can also be quickly removed from the body when the patient's own blood is given back, for example, following hemodilution or from the heart-lung machine in heart surgery.

Colloids, by contrast, go mainly to the vascular space and remain there for longer periods (hours to days). In addition to staying in the vascular space, some, because of their make-up, pull water back from the interstitial to the vascular space. They can, therefore, increase blood volume to a greater amount than the volume of product given. These can also be very useful when edema (excessive water that has moved into the interstitial space) has developed due to the depletion of plasma proteins in major blood loss.

Doctors select the appropriate volume expander or combination of fluids to address the specific needs of the patient. It must be remembered that volume expanders do not carry oxygen like red blood cells do. They simply enable the heart and circulatory system to work more effectively and transport the remaining oxygen-carrying red blood cells around the body. New generation solutions undergoing clinical trials have the ability to provide both volume expansion and oxygen. These have been commonly referred to as "blood substitutes," "synthetic blood" or "oxygen therapeutics." (See Appendix 2)

Fluid Distribution in the Body

40% Solid

60% Water

2/3 Intracellular (within cells)

1/3 Extracellular (outside cells)

25% Intravascular (within blood vessels, in plasma)

75% Interstitial (Outside vessels surrounding cells in the tissue)

Water content of body

Water distribution in body

Extracellular distribution

What is Hemodilution?

Deliberate controlled *hemodilution* is a technique whereby the anesthesiologist uses specific non-blood fluids to dilute the patient's blood. When bleeding occurs, fewer blood cells are actually lost because of its diluted state. There are two ways to do this.

One method, *hypervolemic hemodilution,* infuses fluids into the patient immediately before the operation. The technique both dilutes the patient's blood and expands the volume above normal levels. Furthermore, no blood is removed. The other process, *acute normovolemic hemodilution* — ANH, involves removing some blood from the patient and replacing it with fluids, maintaining normal volume. This allows for a greater degree of dilution than hypervolemic hemodilution.

Acute Normovolemic Hemodilution (ANH)

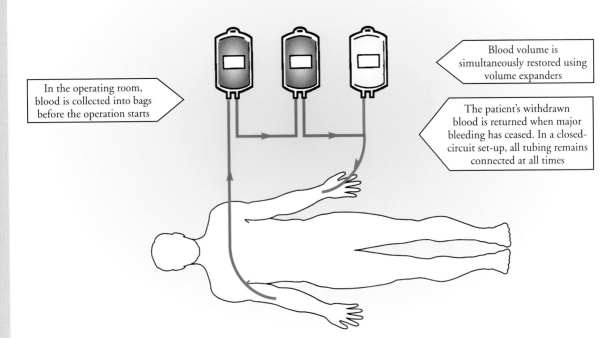

In the operating room, blood is collected into bags before the operation starts

Blood volume is simultaneously restored using volume expanders

The patient's withdrawn blood is returned when major bleeding has ceased. In a closed-circuit set-up, all tubing remains connected at all times

For those seeking bloodless surgery for religious reasons
ANH can be set up in a "closed-circuit" as illustrated

In the operating room, just before the procedure begins, the anesthesiologist draws a predetermined amount of the patient's blood, simultaneously replacing it with a non-blood fluid expander (the withdrawn blood is held in bags). It is important to maintain volume for the heart to work effectively and maintain oxygen delivery to the cells. Hemodilution ensures that whatever blood is lost during the operation has fewer blood cells in it per volume. Because the diluted blood is thinner, it also reduces the load on the heart and allows the blood to flow more easily through the capillaries. Thus oxygen delivery is improved. When major surgical bleeding has stopped, either during or at the end of the operation, the withdrawn supply of the patient's whole blood is returned, still fresh and containing all its platelets and clotting factors.

Hemodilution capitalizes on the body's inbuilt oxygen-carrying reserve and its ability to compensate for and tolerate reduced numbers of red blood cells. This tolerance is further increased by anesthesia. For example, under normal circumstances our cardiovascular system delivers up to four times more than the amount of oxygen consumed by the tissues. Technically, it delivers approximately 1,000 ml of oxygen a minute to the tissues which, in turn, use 200-300 ml a minute. This makes for a large reserve. Along with other mechanisms, the reserve allows our blood to supply all oxygen needs to cells when we are relaxing in a chair. But it can also adapt and supply the dramatically increased needs of strenuous exercise, like running a marathon. During exercise our muscles need more fuel — oxygen. To provide this extra need, the heart beats faster and more efficiently, we breathe more deeply and rapidly, vascular activity increases the blood flow to the muscles and we extract more oxygen from the blood. This ability to compensate also works for us when we lose blood. Even though we have fewer circulating red blood cells, the four-fold reserve mentioned in Chapter 2 along with other compensatory mechanisms allows us to cope. This is particularly so in the controlled environment of the operating room under anesthesia. Just as we use less oxygen when resting, we use even less when asleep. Then our metabolic rate slows even more. Under anesthesia, with sedation, muscle relaxants and our breathing being done for us by the ventilator, our needs are further reduced.

If a person is to undergo an operation that has the potential for major blood loss, more severe hemodilution — taking off more blood — may be possible because of these factors. Some doctors have reported hemodiluting children down to hemoglobin levels between 1 to 3 g/dL in major heart, cancer and spinal surgery.

There are limits to the extent individual patients can be diluted. Adults may not tolerate the levels of hemodilution described for children if hemodilution alone is used. Just as not every person is able to run a marathon, maybe because of heart disease or lack of general fitness, each individual has differing limits of being able to compensate for low blood levels. ANH may not be suitable for patients who have significant coronary artery disease. This, again, would need to be assessed in the preoperative period and hemodilution tailored to the individual and the planned operation. It should also be remembered that hemodilution is just one part of the overall bloodless surgery plan.[3]

However, hemodilution has a number of advantages, not least of all its ability in combination with other techniques to avoid the use of donor blood. It has also been shown to be a more cost-effective alternative to preoperative autologous donation and equal, if not superior, clinically. The following are among its advantages:

- The patient doesn't have to take the time to make regular trips to donate blood.
- Surgery can be scheduled without delay.
- Anemia isn't induced before surgery by the regular donations.
- The blood is not wasted if surgery is cancelled because of illness.
- The risk of giving the patient the wrong blood is eliminated because it never leaves the operating room and, accordingly, does not need testing.
- The blood is fresh and whole, still has all the clotting factors and platelets, isn't subject to the adverse effects of storage and has less chance of bacterial contamination.

Anesthesiologist Dr Thomas Crimi, from Brookdale University Hospital and Medical Center in Brooklyn, New York, reported at the 1999 Hong Kong conference that greater utilization of acute normovolemic hemodilution in combination with other bloodless techniques had brought about the closure of the center's predonation clinic earlier that year. Even though it is a level -1 trauma center, these techniques had reduced blood usage by 75%. He said they had not transfused any patients undergoing prostate removal surgery (radical prostatectomy) for almost two years, an operation which has the potential of very large blood loss, traditionally of one to three liters or more.

ANH has been combined with other techniques to increase its effectiveness. For example, erythropoietin has been used before surgery to increase the patient's hemoglobin level, thus allowing more blood to be withdrawn at the time of surgery. Augmented acute normovolemic hemodilution (AANH™) is a recently emerged term that describes the inclusion of new synthetic oxygen-carrying solutions as the diluent, allowing more extreme hemodilution.

Hypothermia

Hypothermia, or controlled lowering of the body temperature, can be used to reduce a patient's oxygen needs during an operation. It is applied judiciously, though, because it can interfere with coagulation. Following hypothermia, the patient is promptly rewarmed to enable normal clot formation. Hypothermia may have special application for patients who have ruled out any donor blood during major surgical procedures usually associated with massive blood loss. In this event, hypothermia can be used in combination with profound hemodilution and deliberate lowering of blood pressure. This combined technique, however, requires specialists with extensive experience and is performed *only* in specialized medical centers.

Salvaging and Recycling

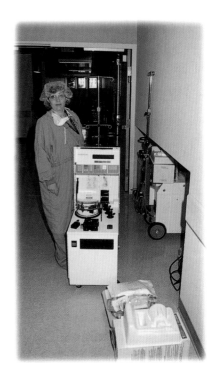

Intraoperative autologous blood salvage is a method used regularly for major procedures in bloodless surgery. Whatever blood is lost through bleeding during an operation is collected and "washed" in what is essentially a high-tech washing machine, commonly known as a "cell saver." The "washing" removes unwanted items such as bits of fat, tissue and possibly bone fragments which are debris from the operation site, and returns mainly the patient's red blood cells. This procedure is quite adequate for most major operations. There is, however, a limit to the amount of blood that can be recycled this way as the process also washes out the blood's clotting factors and removes or damages many of the platelets. Consequently, multiple recycles may lead to coagulation problems.

117

Intraoperative Blood Salvage

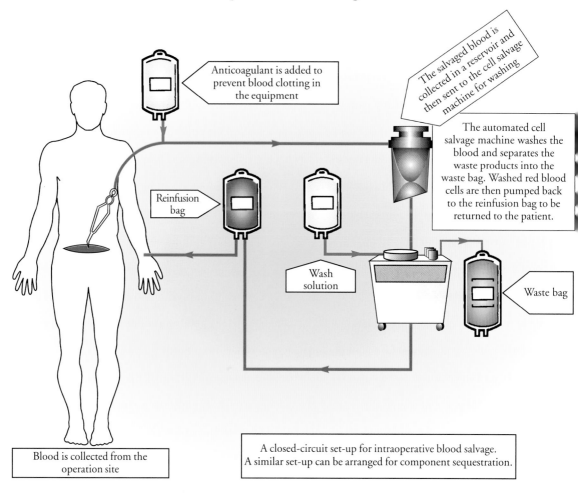

Anticoagulant is added to prevent blood clotting in the equipment

The salvaged blood is collected in a reservoir and then sent to the cell salvage machine for washing

The automated cell salvage machine washes the blood and separates the waste products into the waste bag. Washed red blood cells are then pumped back to the reinfusion bag to be returned to the patient.

Reinfusion bag

Wash solution

Waste bag

Blood is collected from the operation site

A closed-circuit set-up for intraoperative blood salvage. A similar set-up can be arranged for component sequestration.

To overcome this, new techniques and technology have been developed for operations involving large blood loss with multiple recycles by the cell salvage machine. The procedure is known as *component, or, platelet sequestration*. Using the cell salvage machine, some of the patient's blood is removed before the operation begins and platelets and plasma containing clotting factors are separated out and kept in bags. The red cells are returned immediately, with some being kept to facilitate hemodilution when appropriate. As the operation proceeds, the cell salvage machine collects and recycles whatever blood is lost from the operation site. While the red blood cells are being recycled, the collected platelets and coagulation factors are retained for use when needed. On completion of the operation, or when major bleeding is stopped, the collected platelets and clotting factors, along with the initially harvested red cells, are returned. This technique has enabled large blood loss procedures such as liver transplantation and complex heart surgery to be completed without the use of donor blood or blood products.

New cell salvage equipment is constantly being developed and refined. Some of these machines now combine cell salvage with fully automated ANH. Different methods of cell washing, less damaging to the cells, are also being developed. Cell salvage has been used extensively in vascular, orthopedic, cardiac and trauma surgery.

Individually, each of the above procedures can decrease the requirement for blood transfusion. Applied in combination, they have a positive cumulative effect.

> *"Perioperative red cell salvage is technology that is safe, well documented and provides a high-quality product that is safer for the patient than allogeneic blood. The technology should be more widely deployed than at present...This should be an important part of a long-term strategy aimed at protecting and developing the national blood source, both allogeneic and autologous, so that we can cope with the rising demands now and in the future."*

Royal College of Physicians of Edinburgh Consensus Conference on Autologous Transfusion November 1998. Desmond M, et al. Perioperative red cell salvage: a case for implementing the 1995 consensus statement. *Transfusion Medicine* 1999;9:265-268.

Oxygen Support

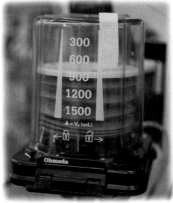

The anesthesiologist is able to manipulate the method and amount of oxygen given the patient during an operation. As described in Chapter 2, while red blood cells carry the bulk of oxygen around the body, there is also a small amount of oxygen dissolved in the plasma (under normal conditions this accounts for about 1.5% of the total oxygen content). Therefore, if more oxygen is required, the anesthesiologist can administer higher concentrations through the ventilator (hyperoxic ventilation), thus allowing more oxygen to be dissolved in the plasma.

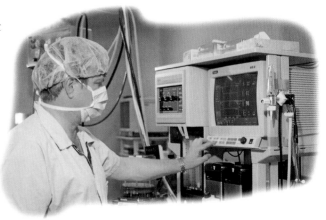

There are limits to this technique but, when used in combination with all the others, it has the cumulative effect of allowing the patient to be managed without blood transfusion. For example, during hemodilution and hypothermia, the dissolved oxygen can constitute 30% of the total blood oxygen content, providing more than half of the body's needs.

Helping the Body to Compensate

Bloodless surgery techniques are all geared to minimizing surgical blood loss so that the patient's hemoglobin never gets to the low levels we have referred to earlier. However, certain strategies need to be employed for patients demanding bloodless management if major blood loss is encountered or has resulted from an emergency.

The changing medical attitude towards blood transfusion is due, in part, to a greater appreciation of physiology. It is now recognized the body has the ability, via a number of natural mechanisms, to compensate for blood loss anemia and maintain oxygen delivery to the tissues. A key factor here is vascular volume (normovolemia). As long as volume is maintained, the body can naturally lift its act.

The heart increases its output of blood by stepping up its pumping rate and the volume of blood moved with each beat. Unless limited by disease, the heart can expand its output five-fold. At the same time, the lungs can expand their loading of oxygen up to 15-fold. Peripheral blood vessels dilate and this, along with the decreased viscosity of the diluted blood, means decreased resistance and increased blood flow to the tissues. Red blood cells release more oxygen from their hemoglobin (remembering the four-fold reserve) and tissues extract more oxygen. Recent work speculates that there may be genetic activity at a cellular level that protects cells during severe anemia. There is still much to be learnt about these processes, which are the subject of concentrated scientific investigation.

There are limits, of course, to the body's natural ability to compensate for low blood levels. When these are reached, many doctors will transfuse. Those adhering to the traditional trigger of 10 g/dL will transfuse well beforehand. More enlightened clinicians, however, have come to appreciate there are other maneuvers which can be used to enhance and augment the body's compensatory mechanisms — aggressive measures which manipulate the body's metabolic rate and further help eliminate the use of blood.

In the controlled environment of the intensive care unit, it is possible to induce a virtual artificial hibernation, dramatically slowing down the body's metabolism. This can reduce the oxygen needs by up to 65%, while high concentrations of oxygen being given via the ventilator ensure each hemoglobin molecule is fully loaded and the dissolved oxygen content maximized. These measures serve to support the body while the blood-building medications work to restore the person's own blood.

However, in certain individuals, these methods are still insufficient to cater for the body's oxygen needs. For those who still do not want blood, one final treatment option is available; *hyperbaric* (high-pressure) *oxygen therapy* (HBO).

Hyperbaric Oxygen Therapy

The hyperbaric oxygen chamber — probably best known for treating divers suffering the bends — exposes the patient to greater atmospheric pressure while he or she is being given high concentrations of oxygen. Under these conditions, the oxygen dissolves more readily into the fluid of the bloodstream.

In bloodless management, the hyperbaric chamber can provide interim life support by supplying the oxygen needs in a situation where the patient has insufficient red blood cells. This, again, buys time for all the blood-building medications to do their work.

Theoretically, a person can survive in a hyperbaric chamber without any blood at all. Under pressure, enough oxygen can be dissolved in blood-replacing fluid to support life. During experiments carried out in 1960, blood was completely removed from pigs and replaced with a volume expander. The pigs were kept alive for some days in the chamber, surviving on the dissolved oxygen. Subsequently, they were reinfused with blood and went about their normal lives. Monitoring over several months showed the animals suffered no apparent harm from their experience.

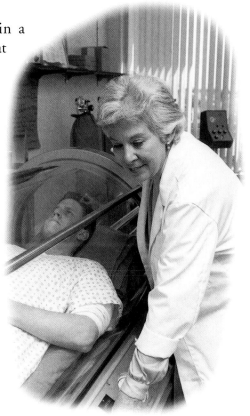

Hyperbaric oxygen has been used successfully to treat patients with severe blood loss and profound anemia. Reports include patients managed with hemoglobins as low as 1 g/dL.

Two cases reported in the journals *Anaesthesia* and *The Journal of the American Medical Association* graphically illustrate the use of HBO therapy.

In Norway, a 55-year-old woman was admitted to hospital suffering from chills, vomiting, jaundice, blood in her urine and low hemoglobin. She was diagnosed as having acute *idiopathic* (of unknown cause) *autoimmune hemolytic anemia.* This is a condition where the body develops antibodies that react against its own red blood cells and destroy them. Despite treatment for the condition, her hemoglobin fell to 3 g/dL, at which time she began to experience symptoms of insufficient oxygen to the brain. Compatible blood could not be found which, even if it had been available, might have worsened her condition. When she deteriorated further, she was transferred to a hyperbaric oxygen chamber at the Royal Norwegian Naval Base in Bergen. After 15 minutes of treatment, her symptoms improved. She underwent intermittent sessions in the chamber for the next five days. By then, her hemoglobin had risen to 5 g/dL and no more HBO treatment was required.

In the UK, a 38-year-old pregnant woman was taken to hospital after experiencing profuse bleeding. Her hemoglobin was 7.4 g/dL. The medical staff assured her that her wish for no blood under any circumstances would be respected. An emergency cesarean section revealed a massive detachment of the placenta and a stillborn baby. During the procedure, there was an estimated blood loss of more than three liters.

Over the next few days, the woman's hemoglobin fell to 2 g/dL and, despite doctors' efforts with all the techniques described earlier in this chapter, she began to experience adverse symptoms from her anemia. This indicated insufficient oxygen supply. Her condition was further complicated by an infection (*staphylococcus aureus*) slowing both her response to erythropoietin therapy and recovery. She was transferred to a hyperbaric chamber where, after the first treatment, the symptoms of severe anemia were reversed. The HBO therapy continued for 16 days, initially three times daily before being reduced to twice a day. Each session lasted 90 minutes. The woman spent a further three weeks in intensive care and thereafter made steady progress. She returned home within three months.

As with all maneuvers, there are potential risks and complications associated with HBO therapy. Pure oxygen is toxic and, when administered for prolonged periods, will cause complications. Hyperbaric physicians are specially trained to avoid and deal with such problems. However, HBO therapy is labor-intensive and costly. For that reason, many doctors consider the therapy a last line of defence — for use in that very rare situation when all else is not enough and blood is either contraindicated, undesirable or unacceptable.

Management of Trauma

The three phases of bloodless surgery discussed earlier have specific application to elective surgery, that is, non-urgent operations, when there is time for planning and preparation of the patient. In an emergency, such as trauma, there is little time for individualized planning. For those who sustain massive acute blood loss in a serious car accident, for example, blood replacement by transfusion (particularly fresh and autologous blood) has been shown to reverse some of the effects of acute blood loss. Consequently, it is still regarded by most doctors as a vital part of treatment.

In general, the management of acute bleeding in emergency patients refusing transfusion requires rapid diagnosis and intervention to control hemorrhage. Physical examination and evaluation, resuscitative measures, and diagnostic procedures are dynamic processes that proceed at the same time.

Management of severe trauma, though, is an extremely challenging field. Some patients die despite all efforts and treatments, including blood transfusion. In such circumstances, questions have been raised about the effects of stored blood on an already compromised body. Similarly, questions are asked about complications of massive transfusion, possibly leading to organ failure, coagulation problems and even death. Reports indicate that the mortality rate after massive transfusion has been typically about 50%. Massive transfusion is defined as more than 10 units of stored whole blood or red cells given within 24 hours.

An alternative measure, using ultrafresh, unrefrigerated whole blood instead of stored blood, is very controversial because the blood is collected immediately from available donors and not tested for diseases. It is also rarely available. Opinions have also changed on how much fluid should be given initially to trauma patients to restore volume before surgery to stop the bleeding is performed.

Complete, lengthy and complex reconstructive surgery (a traditional approach) along with multiple transfusions at a time when the patient is very unstable, can create an irreversible cycle which takes the patient beyond physiological limits. In recent years, a new approach termed "damage control" or "planned reoperation" has been developed to treat hemorrhaging, critically wounded patients with multiple injuries. Initially, the "damage control" strategy uses rapid, temporary methods to stop the bleeding. This is followed by stabilization of the patient in ICU. Reconstructive surgery is performed later after the patient's condition has improved. Simultaneously, this approach has markedly improved the survival rate of patients who have undergone massive trauma. It has also reduced and, in some cases, even eliminated blood transfusions.

Management of trauma patients is undergoing constant review. Those involved in bloodless surgery are seeing some advantages in managing these difficult cases without allogeneic blood. While there is clearly little time for the preoperative preparation, the second two phases of bloodless management, intraoperative and postoperative, are applied aggressively with the prime focus on stopping the bleeding.

A 1992 Netherlands study[4] of major trauma patients set out to discover how low the hemoglobin level could fall in emergencies without increasing the risk of complications. This was at a time when some trauma specialists believed their patients were dying through lack of sufficient transfused blood. The study reviewed 932 consecutive major trauma patients with multiple injuries treated between 1985 and 1990. The medical team compared non-transfused (patients who refused blood for religious reasons) with transfused patients (transfused to the traditional hemoglobin level of 10 g/dL or more). All had sustained large blood loss with hemoglobin levels as low as 2.7 g/dL in the non-transfused group.

The most notable difference between the two groups, apart from very low blood levels in the non-transfused, was that most of the transfused experienced liver failure. This was partially due to the breakdown products of stored blood overloading the liver. While the non-transfused had very low blood levels requiring aggressive management, they all survived. This led the team to the conclusion that low hemoglobin and plasma protein levels did not threaten the patients' chance of survival. In fact, the liver failure seen in the majority of the transfused led to the failure of other organs and death of one of the patients in that group. The study group made this observation: "Not giving blood products to multiple trauma patients seemed to protect them in one way or another from developing severe liver failure."

Since the Netherlands study, other investigators similarly have found that low hemoglobin levels are well tolerated in trauma patients, while liver failure increases with the number of units of blood transfused, leading to higher mortality.

While there are many other reports in medical literature on the subject, a detailed examination of trauma is beyond the scope of this book. Similarly, not covered is the bloodless management of medical problems such as the leukemias and other diseases where blood transfusion has been standard therapy. This area is addressed in bloodless medicine and surgery but, being a subject of its own, is again beyond the scope of this book.

Note: *We have now explored the many techniques and methods that make up the large toolbox of bloodless surgery. Individually, none offers the complete answer for every situation. But when brought together in combination with all the other tools, they contribute to making bloodless surgery most viable. Each tool has its own benefits, risks and limitations. Not all techniques apply to every operation and not necessarily to every patient. Some of the newer equipment and medications may not be readily available in all countries. Substantial costs may be involved in acquiring it. Thus patients will need to discuss with a doctor experienced in bloodless surgery which techniques or combinations of techniques can best be used in their treatment.*

[1] Bloodless surgery is not necessarily dependent on high-tech machines and devices. These are adjuncts and not replacements for good, careful, surgical technique. In fact, many of the bloodless medicine and surgery techniques are relatively simple and inexpensive and so are within the reach of almost any doctor/hospital in the world. This includes those in developing countries where blood transfusions are especially hazardous because of lack of resources for donor screening and blood testing.

[2] Sometimes, if there is uncontrollable bleeding, the surgeon may have to open up the operation site and return to the conventional procedure.

[3] Use of the heart-lung machine in cardiac surgery may dilute the patient's blood too much and, so, techniques are used to avoid excessive hemodilution in these operations.

[4] The study was presented at an international blood transfusion conference in Edinburgh in 1992 by Professor H.J. ten Duis from The Netherlands Groningen University Hospital.

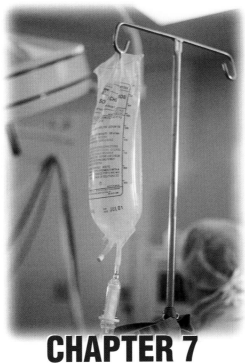

CHAPTER 7

YOU AND BLOODLESS SURGERY: THE FUTURE

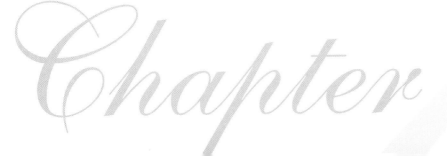

Changing Attitudes and Advancing Techniques

*I*f bloodletting as a medical practice lasted almost 2,500 years, it seems valid to ask: how long will blood transfusion last? Some in the medical profession are adamant it will always be a part of health care. Others predict, just as passionately, it will be obsolete within 10 to 15 years.

Modern transfusions have been standard practice for just on 60 years. Extraordinarily enough, it has only been in the last of those six decades that transfusion's validity as a medical procedure has been examined in any detail at all.

Still, very little is known scientifically about its effectiveness. Only now are the important questions being asked. Do transfusions really work at the tissue level? Do they actually improve the outcome for patients?

The fact is, there has never been a controlled clinical trial that compares transfusion to no transfusion — that is, transfused patients with non-transfused patients. In other words, to this day the efficacy of blood transfusion as a therapy has yet to be scientifically established.

Many experts have emphasized the need for trials to address this gaping issue. The 1999 Canadian TRICC study, discussed in Chapter 4, was the first attempt at a large randomized trial to look at transfusion practice. It was limited, however, in that it simply compared two different transfusion strategies — a liberal policy, on the one hand, and a restrictive one, on the other. It did not examine transfusion versus no transfusion. The study also restricted the scope of its data to critically ill patients in intensive care and this in itself was another major limitation.

Other trials, either under way or being planned, are looking at transfusion thresholds or "triggers." They do not address the basic, unresolved issue.

For many reasons, a randomized clinical trial to determine the fundamental question about transfusion would present extremely difficult ethical issues. Against this, of course, one must ponder the ethical position of those continuing to administer transfusions based on traditions that ignore current scientific evidence.

Traditionally, blood transfusion has been used to treat anemia. Anemia is an abnormal state. While there are in-built reserves and the body is able to compensate for and tolerate, sometimes, even very severe anemia, the condition is associated with risks, complications and reduced physical function. Additionally, it appears that patients with cardiovascular disease are less able to compensate for anemia and may be at increased risk of complications. For decades, banked allogeneic blood has been the major therapy for anemia.

Now, however, questions are being asked about whether anemia is effectively treated this way. At a 1998 meeting of experts to discuss the risks and treatment of perioperative anemia, Dr Jeffrey L. Carson and Dr Arnold Y. Chen, noted how very little evidence existed to support the assumption that transfusions prevented the complications of anemia. Furthermore, they pointed out that very little scientific investigation had been conducted on the effects of anemia on humans. What work that had been undertaken in this area, they contended, showed little benefit accruing from red cell transfusion.

Highlighting the lack of scientific data, they explained they had identified only five published studies between 1956 and 1998 comparing the effects of different transfusion triggers. While none of the studies found any differences in mortality and morbidity between high and low transfusion thresholds, the five studies had involved only a combined total of 207 patients. Consequently, no sound conclusions could be drawn.

However, Dr Carson and his group conducted an extensive, retrospective review of 8,787 elderly patients who required emergency surgery for broken hips, comparing transfused with non-transfused. They found that doctors' transfusion practices varied greatly in patients with hemoglobin levels between 8 and 10 g/dL (80 and 100 g/L). In this group, 56% were given transfusion and had a higher 30-day death rate than the 44% who did not receive a transfusion. After analyzing these data and allowing for patient differences and other variations, they concluded that transfusion had no beneficial effect on either 30-day or 90-day death rates. "We have found no evidence that transfusion improves survival in these elderly hip fracture patients with a high burden of chronic disease and hemoglobin levels greater than 80 g/L. Since there is good evidence about the risks of transfusion, physicians should reconsider whether transfusion is warranted for such patients, keeping in mind the lack of evidence about the possible benefits, such as improving physical function and accelerating recovery after surgery."

When Professor Jean-Francois Hardy and colleagues from the Montreal Heart Institute reviewed 2,661 patients who had undergone heart surgery, they found that postoperative anemia adversely affected complication rates and length of hospital stay. However, they also found that complications and length of stay increased in patients given transfusions to correct their anemia. What is more, such circumstances worsened with the greater number of units given. They reported that there could be a number of interpretations of their results. One was that transfusions were either insufficient or unable to correct inadequate oxygen supply. Another was that the transfusions increased complications, rather than the anemia itself. Disturbingly, patients transfused with the highest hemoglobin levels had the highest incidence of complications and longest hospital stays. Even if this was because they were possibly sicker patients, this would indicate, they said, "that transfusions were, at best, ineffective."

Confirming the lack of evidence for the effectiveness of transfusion, eminent American surgeon Dr Richard Spence commented: "An extensive review of all the relevant clinical literature on transfusion studies, risks and benefits found no conclusive evidence of benefit from red cell transfusion."

Others experts have commented on the fact that it is unknown whether transfused stored blood is able to deliver oxygen to the tissues effectively. The transfused red blood cells pick up oxygen from the lungs and carry it. Still to be comprehended is what happens at tissue level and how effective the red blood cells are in getting to the tissues and delivering their load. The stored cells bind their oxygen more tightly with their membranes becoming less flexible and so less able to squeeze through the tiny capillaries that feed the tissues. They may, in fact, hinder efficient oxygen delivery to the tissues. This could be of particular importance for the critically ill patient.

An editorial in the November, 1999, issue of the journal *Chest* put it succinctly: "It is clear that the transfusion of RBCs may not only *not* help, but may, in fact, do harm to the critically ill patient."

Such findings tend to underline the significance of the words of Dr J.E. Dunphy, emeritus professor of surgery at the University of California School of Medicine, who more than two decades ago wrote in the American College of Surgeons' *Bulletin*: "Transfusion certainly makes the surgeon feel better, but it may not make the patient feel better. Perhaps we all have a tendency to transfuse to make ourselves more comfortable."

"Efficacy of red blood cell transfusions has never been formally evaluated the way drugs and biologics are tested today prior to governmental approval.

"In specific situations with organ dysfunction caused by extreme acute anemia, transfusion of red blood cells has been shown to be an efficacious treatment. In most of these studies, this was achieved by transfusion of fresh, mostly autologous, red blood cells. Large studies have failed to demonstrate an outcome benefit in liberally transfused patients. In contrast, there is strong evidence that liberal transfusion of red blood cells adversely affects morbidity and mortality in surgical and critically ill patients. Judicious and restrictive use of red blood cell transfusion is thus indicated."

Donat R. Spahn (pictured right), Professor of Anesthesiology, Institute of Anesthesiology, University Hospital, Zurich, Switzerland.
Benefits of Red Blood Cell Transfusion: Where is the Evidence?" *Transfusion Alternatives in Transfusion Medicine* 1999;1(1):6-10.

"Data regarding the benefit(s) or efficacy of blood and blood components are largely lacking. Although approximately 12 million units of red blood cells are transfused per year in the United States, the efficacy of this biologic has not been demonstrated in an appropriately controlled, prospective study, nor are there clear criteria by which one would judge the efficacy of red blood cells."

Richard B. Weiskopf MD
More on the Changing Indications for Transfusion of Blood and Blood Components during Anesthesia. Anesthesiology 1996;84(3):498-501.

The Developing Scene

Bloodless surgery takes a proactive approach. It aims either to avoid anemia in the first place by reducing blood loss, or treating the anemia with alternatives to blood transfusion. As discussed, there are already multiple strategies available. The future, it seems, is going to open up even more of these. Presently, developments in bloodless surgery are progressing along a number of lines.

- **Blood substitutes:** One is to produce a so-called artificial blood, or blood substitute — one that has a long shelf-life, does not require matching to the specific patient and one that doesn't transmit infectious diseases. A true "blood substitute," however, will be very difficult to produce because blood, as we have seen, is a complex fluid performing multiple tasks. And so efforts have been directed at developing products that perform the functions of the individual components of blood. For example, to perform the role of the red blood cells, a number of oxygen-carrying substances have been developed. That, in itself, has taken three separate directions: (1) to create synthetic fluids, such as perfluorochemicals, which provide volume expansion and carry oxygen (pictured below, the perfluorochemical, Oxygent being manufactured), (2) to produce synthetically engineered hemoglobin and

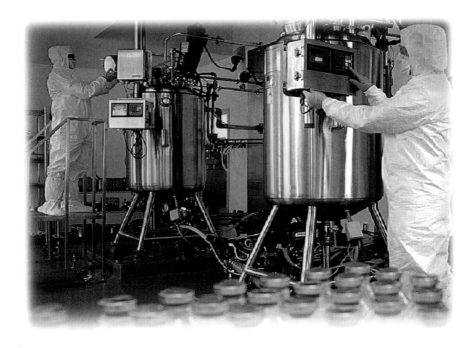

(3) to modify and purify human or animal hemoglobin. All three are currently in clinical trials. If proved safe and effective, these could be used in major surgery or in cases of trauma to carry oxygen temporarily until the body manufactures its own new blood.

Perflubron is the only perfluorochemical in advanced clinical testing. Application for its approval will be filed in the year 2000. Professor Donat Spahn, professor of anesthesiology from University Hospital, Zurich, Switzerland, says: "Once available for clinical medicine, perflubron will completely change transfusion medicine. This will be a revolution in medicine like the introduction of the first antibiotic, penicillin." Professor Spahn, who has been involved with clinical trials using perflubron in Augmented ANH (mentioned in Chapter 6), points to many more applications of this synthetic oxygen carrier. Because of its small particle size – less than one micron in diameter (pictured right) – it could be used for immediate oxygenation of tissues affected, for example, by heart attacks, strokes and other vascular blockages. He sees it having a role in trauma and emergency surgery, decompression sickness and even in improving the preservation of organs for transplantation.

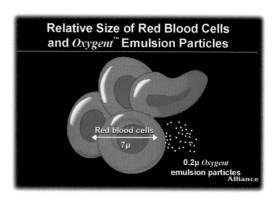

Relative Size of Red Blood Cells and *Oxygent*™ Emulsion Particles

Red blood cells
7μ

0.2μ *Oxygent* emulsion particles
Alliance

Considerable progress is also being made in developing other artificial blood components such as platelets, plasma proteins, clotting factors and immunoglobulins.

- **Blood production stimulants:** Another area of intense investigation has been to produce the factors that stimulate the body to make its own blood. This involves a whole range of developing products, such as synthetic *erythropoietin* (EPO), *thrombopoietin, interleukin-11* and other agents administered to prompt the body to produce the various individual components of blood. "Gene therapy" is yet another area of research. The idea is to stimulate the body's production of its own cell growth substances, like erythropoietin, as well as clotting factors.

Using combinations of the aforementioned, various future scenarios have been painted. For example, in major blood loss procedures, the hemodilution principle could be applied using oxygen-carrying substances to augment oxygen delivery during the operation (pictured below). The maximum amount of the patient's own blood could be withdrawn before the operation starts and replaced with a volume expander. During the operation when blood loss takes place, oxygen delivery would be augmented with the synthetic oxygen carrier. At the completion of the operation, the patient's own blood would be returned (trials have already been carried out using this technique). Or, in the trauma setting, the patient who has lost large volumes of blood could be transfused with these fluids both to restore volume and carry oxygen while surgery is performed to repair the damage. Synthetic platelets and clotting factors could be administered to facilitate clotting, while the blood production stimulating factors would be administered to "rev up" the patient's own blood building factory.

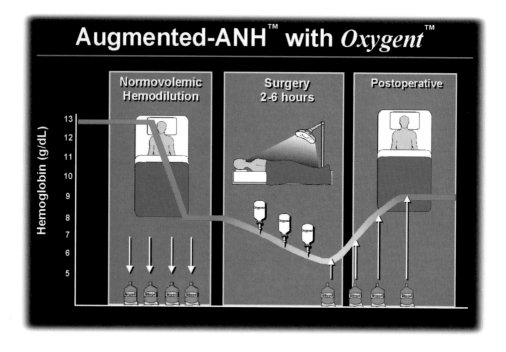

- **Minimally invasive surgery:** The other development has been to modify surgical techniques so that they are less invasive, placing the body under reduced stress and allowing quicker postoperative recovery. Instead of large, open incisions, minimally invasive surgery uses specially designed surgical instruments with lighting and video viewing equipment inserted through very small incisions or natural body openings. A good example is the development of minimally invasive heart surgery (MID CAB – minimally invasive direct CABG; OP CAB – off pump CABG; Heart Port – Endovascular CPB).[1] Traditionally, open-heart surgery has meant a large incision followed by sawing through the breastbone and prising open the ribcage to expose the heart, linking the patient to a heart-lung machine and then stopping the heart. Now, techniques have been developed which allow the surgeon to operate through small incisions or "ports" between the ribs and above the heart. With some techniques, surgery can be performed while the heart is still beating (referred to as "off pump"), avoiding the use of the heart-lung machine. Early reports have already been published on these techniques being applied to patients requiring multiple bypass surgery and valve replacement, with the patients being out of hospital in two or three days. These techniques are designed to reduce pain, scarring and other complications associated with the traditional open approach, thus reducing hospital stay and recovery time. However, not all conditions are suitable for such techniques and these still require traditional open surgery. Additionally, it is still a new procedure and the long-term efficacy is yet to be evaluated.

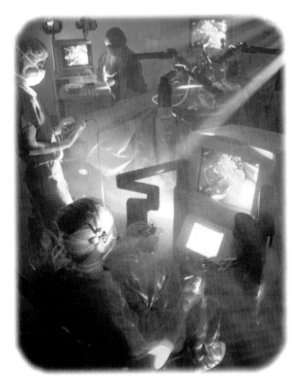

Such advances in minimally invasive, or keyhole surgery, are being taken further with the introduction of even more sophisticated equipment. For example, more recently, a robot has been developed which, positioned above the patient, performs heart surgery through little tubes. Its actions are controlled by the surgeon who could be sitting meters away, or even in an adjoining room. The surgeon commands the robot's instruments by remote control, while watching the patient and the operation site on a TV monitor. The robotic technique reduces human hand movements during a procedure and, consequently, makes for greater precision.

The surgical treatment of life-threatening abdominal aortic aneurysms (ballooning of the large aortic artery in the abdomen) is also undergoing change to a less invasive procedure known as an intra-luminal graft. Whereas it used to be a major operation necessitating a big incision to reach the damaged vessel deep inside the body, now the procedure may be done by inserting a graft or sleeve inside a sheath up through the femoral artery in the groin and positioning it inside the aneurysm. Once positioned, the sheath is removed and the self-expanding graft fills the aneurysm, providing a new channel for the blood. This without transfusion and a blood loss of less than 100ml, or about three or four tablespoons, against the multiple units of transfused blood used in the past.

With these minimally invasive procedures, if all goes well, the patient suffers less blood loss, less trauma, reduced operation time and is out of hospital quicker with shorter recovery period. However, sometimes complications require the surgeon to revert mid-operation to the open procedure. There are many minimally invasive procedures in addition to heart and vascular surgery. These treat various medical conditions covered by the wide fields of general surgery and gastroenterology as well as neurosurgery, obstetrics/gynecology, orthopedics/spinal surgery, thoracic surgery and urology.

Even less invasive procedures such as *stereotactic body radiosurgery* are being used for certain tumors and diseases. These involve no cutting at all and so no bleeding. Instead of using a knife, they fire precisely aimed multiple radiation beams at the lesion. The patient feels nothing, much like having an x-ray or scan. The process uses sophisticated imaging equipment such as CT scans and MRIs combined with computers to map the exact location of the cancer. The equipment then focuses the radiation beams with extreme accuracy on the treatment area. It avoids harming the normal, healthy surrounding tissue — a complication of more conventional radiation treatment methods. These various forms of radiotherapy have been used to treat blood-vessel malformations in the brain, cancers of the brain, neck, chest, abdomen and pelvis, and sometimes tumors which otherwise would be inoperable. (See strategies list on page 153)

The Patient Comes First

All these developments are running in tandem with an increasingly self-assertive demand by the individual in the western world to have more control over life and body. What has been taken for granted in the past is no longer acceptable. The new, questioning mood of better educated communities wants to understand the options, whether offered by the politician, the plumber or the surgeon. It is no longer sufficient to be told what is going to happen. Information, explanation and proper understanding are fast becoming the pre-requisites of acceptance.

The old adage applies in a new medical scenario — the *customer comes first!* People want to be part of the decision-making process with their doctor. No longer are they prepared to be told what to do. Rapidly passing are the days when people said: "You are the doctor, you know best." When something goes wrong with their health, modern patients read and research. In turn, the modern doctor is focusing more on the patient, considering the whole person — their physical, emotional and even spiritual needs and values. More and more patients are saying: "My body, my choice." And more and more doctors are responding.

This growing change of attitude was quietly endorsed in comments by the Australian College of General Practitioners immediately after the tragic news emerged of the Melbourne schoolgirl diagnosed HIV positive in July 1999, several months after undergoing surgery. While it was the first known case in Australia in 15 years of AIDS contracted from contaminated blood, the college made the point that several alternatives to blood transfusions had been developed over the years, including bloodless surgical techniques and blood substitutes. The college spokesman and chair of the West Australian branch, Dr Colin Hughes, said surgeons had a duty of care to explain procedures and options properly to their patients, but were often in too much of a hurry to do so. "The problem has been that the

137

surgeons haven't really explained the patient options nearly as well as they should," he said.

Patients are now forcing change, and bloodless surgery is being patient-driven as more and more request it.

The rapid growth of hospitals worldwide which have established centers for bloodless medicine and surgery, strongly underlines this growing interest in the specialty by both health care professionals and the community. In 1990, there were only five dedicated bloodless surgery centers in the world. Today there are some 200, with numbers continuing to grow. Many are large teaching hospitals performing the full range of specialties, both elective and emergency. As these and other specialist centers grow, doctors are either becoming increasingly involved in the broad concept of bloodless surgery, or, at least, embracing the principles of blood conservation.

Regrettably, scepticism still exists. Much of it is fanned by ignorance. Some doctors believe bloodless surgery is simply restricted to avoiding donor blood use in response to a patient request. Others believe there is no more to it than the use of a cell salvage machine.

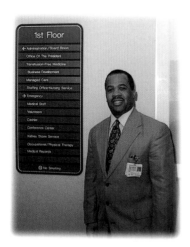

With burgeoning public interest in bloodless surgery, some more opportunistic hospitals unfortunately perceive enticing marketing ploys. As Wayne Henderson[2] (pictured left) put it, "Merely hanging out a shingle in order to attract patients relegates the specialty to the status of inferior or 'second class' medicine, which it clearly is not." This is not bloodless surgery. Bloodless surgery involves much more.

Bloodless medicine and surgery centers have established formal programs to provide top-quality patient care.

Essential to these are a committed hospital administration, personnel to coordinate the programs, and teams of skilled doctors, nurses, technicians and other support staff. Ongoing in-house clinical education is also a key element in a bloodless surgery center, including update lectures and seminars, distribution of the latest clinical research material to staff and doctors and networking with other international specialist centers. This is often done under the direction of a bloodless surgery advisory committee also responsible for quality assurance issues. Access to this treatment is provided through public education lectures, patient hotlines, referral centers and specific admitting policies.

"It is more important to know what sort of person has the disease than what sort of disease the person has."

Sir William Osler, eminent 19th century Canadian physician, researcher, author and teacher.

"Health care recipients have and will become increasingly knowledgeable about risks and benefits of blood transfusion and alternatives to blood transfusions. Physicians increasingly will face patients demanding more information and access to alternatives. Physicians seeking to discharge their obligation to obtain informed consent will be faced with the issue as to what alternatives to allogeneic transfusion must be explained to the patient. The contents and timing of informed consent in relation to blood transfusion will be a legal issue to be determined in the 21st century."

Bonnie Tough LLB, LLM
The Legal Implications of the New Blood System for Health Care Providers and Governments.
In: Huston P, editor. Building a Blood System for the 21st Century. Proceedings and Recommendations. Symposium on blood transfusion and the medical alternatives; 1997 Nov 3-4; Toronto, Canada. Ottawa: Health Canada/Canadian Blood Agency/Canadian Hemophilia Society; 1997:33-34.

How to Access Bloodless Surgery

A telephone call is all you need to do to contact your nearest bloodless surgery or transfusion-free center. The coordinator, after assessing your needs, will refer you to the appropriate specialists available in the hospital team.

Sometimes, the type of surgery you require may not be performed in your local bloodless surgery center. Costs and the demands of

139

specialization remain the primary inhibiting factors. That being so, the staff will put you in touch with the most conveniently located team able to handle your needs.

Many cities and regions do not have the dedicated bloodless surgery centers as we have described in this book. There are, however, specialist doctors and surgeons in hospitals throughout the world who have an interest and are involved in bloodless surgery techniques. In such circumstances, patients may need to ask their family physician as the first point of contact to find a surgeon in the area who understands bloodless surgery. Unfortunately, many family doctors are still unfamiliar with bloodless surgery and you may need to seek the assistance of your local hospital administration or the health authority in the district. The next step is to discuss with the surgeon and anesthesiologist his or her experience with blood conservation techniques and which of these they will be utilizing in your management. Should the surgeon or anesthesiologist be reluctant to go ahead, it may then be advisable to ask to be referred to another clinician experienced in performing an operation according to the patient's wishes. Specialists at bloodless surgery centers are always willing to be consulted and provide information to treating doctors.

In short, depending on the circumstances and the availability of bloodless surgery services in the city or region where the prospective patient lives, it may require shopping around to make the right contacts. If one doctor can't help, another will.

There are also several bloodless surgery sites on the Internet with the latest news on research and development. Depending on the country of abode and the type of surgery, the final decision may necessitate travelling overseas for an operation. We would draw your attention to the list of bloodless surgery centers at the back of this book (Appendix 3).

Those contemplating elective surgery should keep in mind the fundamental concepts of bloodless medicine during discussions with their doctor or specialist. They will then be in a better position to decide to what extent they are prepared to expose themselves to any possible risk associated with transfused blood. They may well agree to accept limited transfusion if, at some point their doctor believes it to be necessary. In this situation they may still demand that the correct bloodless surgery techniques are applied and everything possible is done to avoid donor blood.

Others may decide they will refuse blood from another person under all circumstances. In this event, they will outline to their doctors the acceptable alternative techniques. This, enables the doctor to plan their treatment accordingly. Both patient and doctor should come to a clear, mutual agreement on the treatment plan. This should be documented in the medical records and conveyed to all members of the treating team. Once an agreement has been made and documented, doctors and hospitals are ethically and legally bound to abide by the patient's wishes.

Wanted: Better Education

The medical profession's caution towards new developments has made it generally slow to move away from entrenched practices and to embrace new approaches. Such has been the case with what has become a traditional, albeit comparatively recent, reliance on blood transfusion.

Bloodless surgery as such is not yet taught in medical schools.[3] Indeed, until recently, the whole subject of blood transfusion has had little attention in medical schools. Back in 1965, Dr Louis Diamond wrote, "Few medical school curricula and rare residency training programs or postgraduate courses contain lectures on transfusion practices and the proper materials to use in specific situations. As a result, blood is often used wastefully, improperly, and dangerously." In 1998, the British Medical Journal publication, *ABC of Transfusion*, indicated by its comments that there was still a lot of room for improvement: "The essentials of blood transfusion are still not adequately covered in the curriculum of most medical schools. Not infrequently, a houseman (a recent medical graduate at a hospital) will be called on to administer a blood component without knowing how to do it." Surveys have shown that even many specialists are not well informed on both the risks of transfusion and indications for its use.

"We found widespread deficiencies in physicians' knowledge of transfusion risks and indications. Each transfusion risk was estimated correctly by fewer than half of the physicians surveyed, and only 31% responded correctly to a set of four questions regarding transfusion indications. Attending physicians routinely had lower

knowledge scores than did residents, yet they exhibited more confidence in their knowledge. Residents' transfusion decisions, however, were strongly influenced by the desires of their attending physicians, resulting in their ordering potentially inappropriate transfusions. Of the residents surveyed, 61% indicated that they ordered transfusions that they judged unnecessary at least once a month because a more senior physician suggested that they do so."

Salem-Schatz SR, et al. Influence of Clinical Knowledge, Organizational Context, and Practice Style on Transfusion Decision Making: Implications for Practice Change Strategies. *The Journal of the American Medical Association* 1990;264(4):476-483.

"Variation in the practice of the administration of blood is becoming increasingly evident from audit, both local and national . . . There are no recognized guidelines on which to base local procedures for the ordering and administration of blood and the management of transfused patients."

British Committee for Standards in Haematology, Blood Transfusion Task Force in collaboration with the Royal College of Nursing and the Royal College of Surgeons of England. The administration of blood and blood components and the management of transfused patients. *Transfusion Medicine* 1999;9:227-238.

Whither Bloodless Medicine and Surgery?

Dr Aryeh Shander believes conservative thinking should be balanced with an open mind for advancement. He says: "Clinical medicine is an art that looks for science to confirm and improve the observations of most if not all physicians. The approach to the patient who needs blood is based on old patterns of care that were applicable years ago. As our knowledge of the risk of transfusion is confirmed by science and the corresponding knowledge of the increasing lack of efficacy of allogeneic blood is increasing, physicians have no choice but to employ known alternatives and look for new ways to deliver this care."

Heart surgeon Manuel Estioko, says: "The better informed public equates to better patients who will be requesting and expecting more quality care without blood transfusion. The future of the specialty of bloodless medicine and surgery is bright. I predict that transfusion-free concepts will be embraced by more physicians in their practices in all specialties; will be incorporated in medical school curricula, in residency programs, and postgraduate training."[4] He also predicts that in the near future there may be a Specialty Board to provide certification for doctors in transfusion-free medical care.

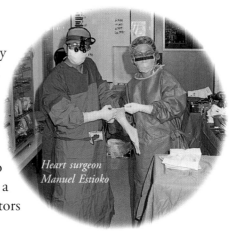

Heart surgeon Manuel Estioko

Wayne Henderson, manager of the Transfusion-Free Medicine and Surgery Center, Good Samaritan Hospital, Los Angeles, forsees a major turnaround in attitudes towards bloodless surgery. He told the authors: "The result of medical approaches like transfusion-free medicine is that the time will come when patients will be able to request this service from any medical facility where they might seek treatment. Transfusion-free medicine will become synonymous with appropriate medical care. Then, the questions will not be, 'is there any reason you object to receiving a blood transfusion?' but rather, 'is there any reason why you would accept a transfusion?' Clearly, education is the key in order for the principles of transfusion-free care to be disseminated on the widest possible scale. This should be done in medical and nursing schools alike, with the emphasis on a consultative rather than a paternalistic approach to patient care."

According to Professor Ciril Godec,[5] speaking in Chicago in 1998, bloodless surgery is no longer an obscure specialty. "Bloodless medicine and surgery is a driving force in the practice of medicine today." In a subsequent newspaper article written the same year, Professor Godec made the observation: "It is quite possible that in the very near future transfusion will be eliminated altogether...Transfusion is not only costly and dangerous; it simply does not provide the highest quality of care that the patient deserves."

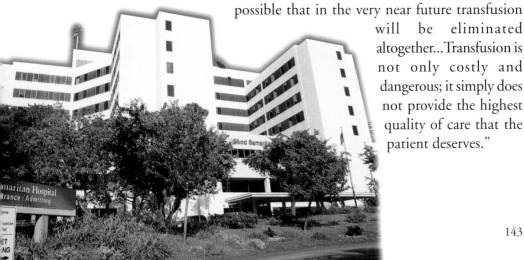

Dr Aryeh Shander regards the future for bloodless medicine and surgery in the short, mid and long terms. "Short-term," he says, "is to continue to educate doctors and make all aware of current treatments and help them rethink their habits. Mid-term, is the full development of genetically engineered factors of blood that are cost efficient, including acceptable oxygen carriers. Long-term is establishing the fact that allogeneic transfusions are a thing of the past and will never be seen again in medicine!"

A VISION OF THE FUTURE

Dr Richard K Spence (pictured right), a highly respected authority on bloodless medicine and surgery, has written this special account for Your Body, Your Choice, summarizing the progress of bloodless surgery and looking to its future.

Dr Spence has been Chief of Surgery, Staten Island University Hospital, New York, and Visiting Professor of Surgery at State University of New York Health Sciences Center. His most recent appointments are Director, Alabama Center for Transfusion Alternatives and Director of Surgical Education for the Baptist Health Systems Hospitals.

Certified in both general and vascular surgery and a Fellow of the American College of Surgeons, Dr Spence is an active member of numerous local, national and international societies. He is immediate past president of the Association for Surgical Education and has served on the board of the National Association of Bloodless Medicine and Surgery.

A founding member of NATA, the Network for the Advancement of Transfusion Alternatives, Dr Spence is considered to be one of the founders of bloodless medicine and surgery as a discipline. He has written extensively, with more than 200 abstracts, individual articles and book chapters to his name. He is a much sought-after speaker internationally and serves as a consultant with several industry leaders in bloodless medicine and surgery.

The basic tenets of bloodless medicine and surgery — avoiding blood loss and doing no harm while performing the best surgery possible — have been a part of sound surgical practice since the first surgeon walked into the first

144

operating room. Similarly, it has been recognized since Blundell performed the first human to human transfusion in 1818 that allogeneic blood transfusion was a hazardous business. The risks may have changed from ABO incompatibility to transmission of the hepatitis C virus, but they remain equally as lethal. Recognition of this lethal risk in the form of transfusion-transmitted AIDS in the 1980s was a wake-up call for medicine. Individual physicians began to look for answers to the problem. Encouragement from those seeking alternatives to blood for religious reasons, along with the introduction of the first blood substitutes, led to the development of fledgling centers where patients refusing blood transfusion could be treated safely and effectively. Physicians re-learned the lessons of the past, questioned traditional transfusion practices and spurred on the development of new methodologies through cooperative efforts with transfusion specialists in a wide variety of fields. These efforts led to the establishment and proliferation of bloodless medicine and surgery centers around the world.

Where are we now and where are we going? Bloodless medicine and surgery has become a well-established focus in modern medical practice. Some hospitals use it primarily as a marketing scheme to gain more patients; most see it as sound medical practice that leads to better patient care. The discipline crosses multiple borders as witnessed by the interest and involvement of medical practitioners of all specialties, attorneys, administrators, legislators, the religious community and the lay public. Through their efforts, bloodless medicine and surgery has evolved into a broader understanding, or a medical philosophy that seeks to employ appropriate transfusion alternatives for all patients, not just those who wish "bloodless" surgery. These alternatives are far ranging and include hemodilution, predonation of blood, autotransfusion, drugs that limit blood loss or restore red cell mass, modification of both transfusion triggers and surgical techniques and the use of leukoreduced allogeneic blood when it is necessary. Not only patients have benefited from this work. Medical textbooks are being re-written as the basics of transfusion science and practice are re-examined in light of our new understanding.

So, it would seem that much progress has been made in the field of bloodless medicine and surgery. There are some 200 centers around the world, we have an international forum for the exchange of ideas — NATA, or the Network for the Advancement of Transfusion Alternatives — and a brand new journal, *Transfusion Alternatives in Transfusion Medicine.* We are proving that bloodless medicine and surgery not only is sound medical practice but also is cost-effective. Clinical trials of blood substitutes and transfusion practices are underway. These are noteworthy accomplishments and are worthy of our collective pride in a job well done. However, we should not be content with the status quo. We need to continue our cooperative efforts at seeking out the information and methods we need to make us even better physicians. We must continue to monitor our own efforts and to share our data as a source of learning. Education is paramount. At present, much of what we preach is being heard only by the choir. We must strive to get our message out to the broader medical and lay communities.

I believe we risk failure if we continue to identify ourselves as a niche or a form of "boutique" medicine that is applicable only to select groups of patients. The lessons we have learned and teach must spread beyond individual centers of excellence. The age-old tenets of bloodless medicine and surgery and our refinements to them must be taught to all physicians as a part of basic medical education that emphasizes benefit over risk in our treatment philosophies. Only after we have accomplished this will a patient be able to walk into any hospital in the world with the comfort of knowing that safe transfusion practices are accepted standards. I see a future where a bloodless medicine and surgery center is a thing of the past, having been replaced by the universal practice of transfusion alternatives.

1   CABG = coronary artery bypass graft, CPB = cardiopulmonary bypass.
2   Henderson, Wayne M. Jr., Manager, Transfusion-Free Medicine & Surgery Center, Good Samaritan Hospital, Los Angeles, California, speaking at the 3rd Transfusion-Free Medicine & Surgery International Conference, Los Angeles, California, September 11-12, 1998.
3   Some large bloodless surgery centers (such as the Transfusion-Free Medicine and Surgery Center, Good Samaritan Hospital, Los Angeles California) are considering the development of post-graduate schools.
4   Estioko, Dr Manuel R., cardiovascular and thoracic surgeon, speaking on the subject "Quality Patient Care - The Goal of Bloodless Medicine and Surgery" at the Bloodless Medicine and Surgery International Conference – Strategies to Avoid Blood Transfusions II, Los Angeles 1996.
5   Godec, Dr Ciril, Professor of Clinical Urology at State University of New York, speaking at the Chicago Bloodless Medicine and Surgery Conference in 1998.

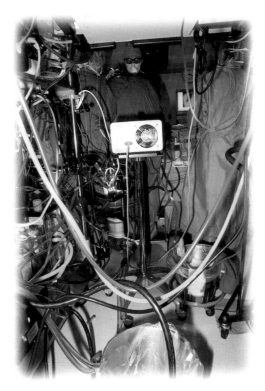

APPENDICES

Appendices

APPENDIX I

TRANSFUSION RISKS AND COMPLICATIONS

Immediate Immune Reactions

- **Acute hemolytic transfusion reaction**
  The most severe immediate immune reaction is referred to as *acute hemolytic* (red cell disintegration or breakdown) *transfusion reaction*. While this can result from undetected incompatibilities in the grouping and cross-matching, the most common cause is the wrong blood type (ABO incompatibility) being given to a person, almost always a result of human clerical error. Blood passes through many hands before being given to the person and, although rare, mistakes can be made. In 1996, it was reported that wrong blood is given to the wrong patient as much as once in every 12,000 transfusions. This mistake can result in death. A 1976-1985 report on transfusion showed that 58% of identified transfusion deaths were caused by this type of hemolytic reaction.

  Estimates of the incidence of this transfusion reaction range from 1 in every 19,000 units transfused to 1 in 33,000. Those resulting in death are estimated to be between 1 in 250,000 to 1,000,000 units.

- **Febrile reactions (estimated risk – 1 in 50 units)**
  The most common immediate reaction is referred to as *febrile* (fever) reaction. This usually happens when the patient's white blood cell antibodies react with the donor's white cells. Additionally, it has been suggested "debris" from cell breakdown in storage may contribute. Common symptoms are fever, chills, headache, muscle pain and nausea. Reports have suggested that anywhere between 1% and 34% of transfused patients experience some sort of febrile reaction. Although not life-threatening, this complication adds significantly to the cost of patient care.

- **Transfusion-related acute lung injury (estimated risk – 1 in 5,000 units)**
  This reaction appears to be caused by white cell antibody/antigen reactions and possibly other transfusion complications. Fluid develops on the lungs (*pulmonary edema*) and in severe cases the person may suffer fever, chills, low

blood pressure and cyanosis (bluish discoloration of the skin caused by oxygen shortage). With treatment, it is estimated that about 90% of patients recover.

- **Allergic reactions (estimated risk – minor reactions 1 in 100 units; anaphylactic shock 1 in 500,000 units)**
  Allergic reactions to proteins in the transfused blood and other facets of the immune system range from mild and common, causing a raised reddish itching rash on the skin (*urticaria*) and sometimes fever, chills and wheezing, to rare but very severe and fatal. Severe allergic reactions (anaphylaxis) manifest in profound low blood pressure, labored breathing, pulmonary edema and respiratory and heart arrest. Severe allergic reactions require immediate aggressive treatment because of very high mortality rates.

Delayed Immune Reactions

- **Delayed hemolytic transfusion reactions (estimated risk – 1 in 500 units)**
  Other less serious forms of hemolytic reactions can appear in a delayed form days to months after the transfusion when white cells or developed antibodies attack the red blood cells. The patient may become anemic, develop mild jaundice, fever and impaired kidney function. On rare occasions this reaction can be severe and even fatal.

- **Graft-versus-host disease (estimated risk – rare, possibly 1 in 750,000 units)**
  Another serious but rare immune reaction is graft-versus-host disease. This occurs when the donor's blood (graft) mounts an immune response against a recipient (host). Although rare, this complication is often fatal despite treatment.

- **Post-transfusion purpura (estimated risk – rare)**
  In rare cases, platelet antibodies in the transfusion destroy the recipient's platelets. Lowered platelet levels (*thrombocytopenia*) may manifest as purple areas on the skin (*purpura*) caused by bleeding into the skin, and can increase the risk of severe hemorrhage. The condition often resolves, but sometimes treatment is necessary because it can be fatal.

- Immune suppression (estimated risk – potentially 1 in 1 units)
  As described earlier, transfusions suppress or modify many facets of the immune system, possibly for the long term. This area is undergoing serious investigation because, whereas other complications listed here have a varying occurrence risk in the number of units transfused, immune suppression may be a one-in-one risk.

Non-Immune Reactions and Complications

Listed among the non-immune reactions are infectious diseases as described earlier. Other non-immune complications are as follows:

- Non-immune hemolysis (estimated risk – rare)
  May be caused if the blood is mixed with the wrong fluids or subjected to freezing or overheating.

- Bacterial contamination (estimated risk – 1 in 25,000 units)
  During the collection, storage and handling process blood can be contaminated with bacteria such as *yersinia*. While improved processing has reduced the incidence of this, when it does occur it is a very severe reaction and can result in death.

- Microaggregates (estimated risk – unknown)
  During storage, small clots form along with clumps of fibrin, platelets, white cells, cell fragments and other degenerative products (*microaggregates*). When transfused these can pass through standard blood filters and impair blood flow through the capillaries. Some have suggested *microaggregates* can contribute to lung damage and activation of the coagulation system. They may also stimulate other untoward responses in the body's immune and defense systems. There are special microfilters which can remove *microaggregates*, but these are not routinely used.

- Circulatory overload (estimated risk – 1 in 10,000 units)
  Transfusion given either too rapidly, or to small children, the elderly or patients with kidney or heart problems may result in an overloading of the body's circulatory system. This in turn causes an accumulation of fluid in the lungs, decreased oxygen delivery to parts of the body and, in severe cases, heart failure.

- **Coagulation disturbances (estimated risk – unknown)**
  Massive transfusions can dilute platelets and coagulation factors to the point where the blood's ability to clot is compromised, contributing to continued bleeding. Further disturbances to the coagulation system may be caused by breakdown products in old stored blood, creating additional bleeding problems.

- **Iron overload (estimated risk – unknown)**
  This is usually only a problem for patients receiving repeated transfusions over a prolonged period. As explained earlier, red blood cells contain iron. Repeated transfusions create an accumulation of iron. At excessive levels iron can become toxic, damaging the liver, heart, pancreas and organs of the endocrine system.

- **Metabolic complications (estimated risk – unknown)**
  Blood in storage is quite a different product to the blood in our veins. When blood is stored in the refrigerator in a sealed plastic bag with anticoagulant and preservatives added, it undergoes a number of chemical changes. For example, stored blood becomes acidic (normal blood is slightly alkaline) and develops elevated levels of sodium, glucose, potassium and ammonium. Reactions to these chemical changes can create an extra load on the critically ill patient.

  Stored blood is cold (approximately 4 °C). If large amounts are given and not warmed correctly, the blood can lower the body temperature (hypothermia) and cause heart rhythm problems.

- **Compromise of oxygen transport (estimated risk – unknown)**
  In storage, red blood cells lose their energy supply (*ATP*). Consequently, they lose their flexibility and form, changing from a bi-concave disc to a more rigid sphere shape, making them less able to squeeze their way through the narrow capillaries to deliver their load of oxygen to the cells. Additionally, stored red cells lose a substance known as 2,3-DPG, a molecule which regulates the hemoglobin's ability to pick up, hold onto and release its load of oxygen. Reduced 2,3-DPG levels mean oxygen binds more tightly to the hemoglobin, resulting in less oxygen being released to the cells. So the transfused stored red blood cells are impaired in their vital role of delivering oxygen to the cells, the very reason for which they are transfused. 2,3-DPG levels in the

transfused blood appear to begin being restored within two to four hours of being within the body, but may not return to normal levels for 24 hours or even longer.

Other changes to the hemoglobin while in storage further contribute to this problem. One textbook suggests that stored blood contains as much as 13.8% abnormal hemoglobin and, when transfused, can cause *hypoxia* (a lack of oxygen to the tissues) and impaired cardiovascular function in critically ill patients.

- **Depression of erythropoiesis (estimated risk – frequent)**
  The transfused blood can suppress or turn off the body's normal signal system to produce more blood (*erythropoiesis*). Consequently when the transfused cells are finally removed from the system by the body's natural processes (approximately three months), the patient can be left with a lower hemoglobin level than before the transfusion was given.

- **Multi-organ failure**
  Some investigators have reported that when patients are transfused with large amounts of old stored blood there is an increased incidence of multi-organ failure. This has been suggested to be related to the degenerative and breakdown products in stored blood.

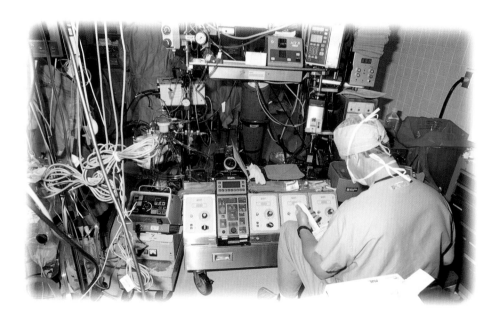

APPENDIX 2

BLOODLESS MEDICINE & SURGERY STRATEGIES

SURGICAL DEVICES/EQUIPMENT FOR MINIMIZING BLOOD LOSS:[1,2,3,4,5,6]

Electrocautery[7]
Electrosurgery
Laser surgery[8]
Argon beam coagulator[9,10,11]
Ultrasonic scalpels[12]
Hemostatic microwave scalpels[13,14,15]
Water jet dissector[16,17]
Cryosurgery[18]
Radiotherapy [19,20,21,22,23] (eg. conformal radiotherapy, gamma knife radiosurgery, intensity-modulated radiotherapy (IMRT), stereotactic body radiosurgery)

SURGICAL AND ANESTHETIC TECHNIQUES TO MINIMIZE BLOOD LOSS:[24,25,26,27]

Preoperative assessment, workup and planning[28,29,30,31]
Careful management of anticoagulation[32,33]
Meticulous hemostasis - careful, gentle dissection along avascular anatomical planes[34]
Mechanical occlusion of bleeding vessel[35,36]
Local vasoconstrictive agents[37,38,39]
Arterial embolization[40,41,42]
Minimally invasive surgery - endoscopic/laparoscopic surgery [43,44,45,46]
Enlarged surgical team - minimal time[47,48,49]
Patient positioning[50,51,52]
Staging complex procedures[53]
Tourniquet[54,55]
Hypotensive anesthesia / controlled deliberate hypotension[56,57]
Induced hypothermia - in special situations[58,59]
Maintenance of normothermia during the intraoperative and postoperative period[60,61]
Autotransfusion:[62]
    Preoperative autologous blood donation (PABD)[63]
    Acute normovolemic hemodilution (ANH)[64,65,66,67,68,69,70]
    Augmented acute normovolemic hemodilution
    Hypervolemic hemodilution[71,72]
    Intraoperative blood salvage[73,74,75,76,77,78]
    Autologous component / platelet sequestration[79,80,81,82]
    Postoperative blood salvage[83,84,85]
Control or minimize hemodilution in cardiac surgery[86,87,88]

Appropriate oxygen support[89],[90]

Pharmacological agents to reduce bleeding[91],[92]

MONITORING DEVICES AND TECHNIQUES TO LIMIT IATROGENIC BLOOD LOSS:[93]

Transcutaneous oxygen monitor

Pulse oximeter

Pediatric microsampling tubes[94],[95]

Point-of-care whole blood microsampling[96]

Multiple tests per sample – careful planning (liaise with laboratory and clinical pharmacist)[97]

SYNTHETIC VOLUME EXPANDERS:[98],[99],[100],[101],[102]

Crystalloids:

Sodium chloride injection solutions
   (isotonic or hypertonic saline)

Compound sodium lactate solutions
   (Hartmann's Solution, Lactated
   Ringer's injection)

Glucose (dextrose) injection solutions

Colloids:

Gelatins
   Succinylated gelatin
   Dialdehyde cross-linked gelatin
   Di-isocyanate urea-linked gelatin
   (eg. polygeline)

Starches
   Pentastarch
   Hetastarch
   Low molecular weight starches
   Dextrans
   (consider pretreatment with dextran
   1 to reduce anaphylaxis risk[103])

HEMOSTATIC AGENTS:[104],[105]

Antifibrinolytic / hemostatic drugs:

Aminocaproic acid[106],[107],[108]

Tranexamic acid[109],[110],[111],[112],[113]

Aprotinin[114],[115],[116],[117],[118],[119]

Vasoconstrictor / procoagulant drugs:

Desmopressin[120],[121]

Vasopressin[122],[123]

Conjugated estrogens[124],[125]

Norethisterone (norethindrone)[126],[127]

Medroxyprogesterone[128]

Vitamin K[129]

Topical Hemostatic Agents:[130]

Microfibrillar collagen

Microfibrillar collagen hemostat spray

Absorbable collagen

Collagen fleece

Absorbable gelatin sponge

Absorbable oxidized cellulose

Thrombin

Bone wax

Tissue Adhesives[131],[132],[133],[134],[135]

Autologous fibrin glue[136],[137]

Autologous platelet gel[138]

THERAPEUTIC AGENTS AND TECHNIQUES FOR MANAGING SEVERE ANEMIA:[139]

Minimize blood loss

Stop the bleeding!
  Prompt reoperation to stop bleeding
Avoid hypertension[146]
Restrict volume and frequency of
  blood sampling
Blood salvage
Maintain normothermia unless
  hypothermia is indicated
Hemostatic agents

Maximize oxygen delivery[163,164]

Maintain intravascular volume[165,166,167]
Maintain cardiovascular support[168,169,170]
Ventilatory and oxygen support[171,172]
Hyperbaric oxygen therapy[173,174,175]

Minimize oxygen consumption[186,187]

Appropriate analgesia
Sedation and paralysis
Hypothermia - with caution
Mechanical ventilation

Maximize blood production

Iron (oral or i.v.)[140,141,142,143,144]
Vitamin C[145]
Epoetin alfa
  (EPO)[147,148,149,150,151,152,153,154,155,156,157]
Folic acid[158]
Vitamin B12[159]
Anabolic steroids[160,161]
Nutritional support (oral or i.v.)[162]
Other hematopoietic factors
  (e.g., IL-11, G-CSF)

**Manage immunologic /
hematalogic disorders**

Immunosuppressive agents if indicated

Acceptance of lower hemoglobin levels

10/30 rule has no scientific
  basis[176,177,178,179,180,181,182,183,184,185]

Other considerations

Avoid infections / treat promptly if
  develop
Consider drug interactions that may
  increase anemia or bleeding
Edema formation from large volumes of
  crystalloid

RECOMBINANT HUMAN HEMATOPOIETIC GROWTH FACTORS:
(Promoting blood formation)

Generic name	Approved name(s)	Stimulates formation of
Erythropoietin (EPO)	epoetin alfa	red blood cells
Granulocyte colony-stimulating factor (G-CSF)[188,189]	filgrastim, lenograstim	specific types of white blood cells
Granulocyte-macrophage colony-stimulating factor (GM-CSF)[190]	molgramostim, sargramostim	specific types of white blood cells
Interleukin-11 (IL-11)[191,192,193]	oprelvekin	platelets
Thrombopoietin (TPO)[194,195] *	thrombopoetin	platelets (also red cells?)
Stem cell factor (SCF)[196] *	ancestim	stem cells (enhances effect of other factors)

RECOMBINANT CLOTTING FACTORS:

Factor VIIa
Factor VIII
Factor IX

OXYGEN-CARRYING SOLUTIONS:[197, 198, 199, 200]

Perfluorochemicals *
Recombinant human hemoglobin *
Human-derived hemoglobin-based oxygen carriers *
Animal-derived hemoglobin-based oxygen carriers *

Products marked with an asterisk are currently undergoing clinical trials.

References for Bloodless Medicine and Surgery Strategies

1   Spence RK. Transfusion and Surgery. *Current Problems in Surgery.* 1993;XXX(12):1103-1180
2   Spence RK. Blood saving strategies in surgical patients. In: Petz LD, Swisher SN, Kleinman S, et al, editors. *Clinical Practice of Transfusion Medicine.* Third edition. New York: Churchill Livingstone; 1996. p. 521-537.
3   Cooley DA. Conservation of blood during cardiovascular surgery. *Am J Surg* 1995;170(6A suppl):53S-59S.
4   Nelson CL, Fontenot J. Ten strategies to reduce blood loss in orthopedic surgery. *Am J Surg* 1995;170(6A suppl):64S-68S.
5   Sculco TP. Blood Management in Orthopedic Surgery. *Am J Surg* 1995;170(6A suppl):60S-63S.
6   Spence RK. Surgical red blood cell transfusion policies. *Am J Surg* 1995; 170(6A suppl):3S-15S.
7   Atabek U, Spence RK, Pello M, et al. Pancreaticoduodenectomy without homologous blood transfusion in an anemic Jehovah's Witness. *Arch Surg* 1992;127:349-351.
8   Grobbelaar AO, Horlock N, Gault DT. Gorlin's syndrome: the role of the carbon dioxide laser in patient management. *Ann Plast Surg* 1997;39(4):366-367
9   Ward PH, Castro DJ, Ward S. A significant new contribution to radical head and neck surgery. The argon beam coagulator as an effective means of limiting blood loss. *Arch Otolaryngol Head Neck Surg* 1989;115(8):921-3.
10 Dunham CM, Conwell EE, Militello P. The role of the argon beam coagulator in splenic salvage. *Surg Gynecol Obstet* 1991;173(3):179-82.
11 Cooley DA. Conservation of Blood During Cardiovascular Surgery. *Am J Surg* 1995;170(suppl 6A):53S-59S.
12 Rees M, Plant G, Wells J, et al. One hundred fifty hepatic resections: evolution of technique towards bloodless surgery. *Br J Surg* 1996;83(11):1526-29.
13 Reed WP, Taylor LS. The microwave coagulating scalpel: Clinical use. *Contemp Surg* 1990; 36(6):22-5.
14 Stauffer UG. The Shaw haemostatic scalpel in paediatric surgery: clinical report on 3000 operations. *Prog Pediatr Surg* 1990;25:39-47
15 Zhou XD, Tang ZY, Yu YQ, et al. Microwave surgery in the treatment of hepatocellular carcinoma. *Semin Surg Oncol* 1993;9(4):318-322.
16 Baer HU, Stain SC, Guastella R, et al. Hepatic resection using a water jet dissector. *HPB Surg* 1993;6:189-198.
17 Spence RK. Emerging Trends in Surgical Blood Transfusion. *Seminars in Hematology* 1997;34(3):48-53

18 Bilchik AJ, Sarantou T, Wardlaw JC, Ramming KP. Cryosurgery causes a profound reduction in tumor markers in hepatoma and noncolorectal hepatic metastases. *Am Surg* 1997;63(9):796-800.

19 Dearnaley DP, Khoo VS, Norman AR, et al. Comparison of radiation side-effects of conformal and conventional radiotherapy in prostate cancer: a randomised trial. *Lancet* 1999;353:267-272.

20 V'arady P, Dheerendra P, Ny'ary I, et al. Neurosurgery using the Gamma Knife. *Orv Hetil* 1999;140(7):331-345.

21 Kondziolka D, Lunsford LD, McLaughlin MR, Flickinger JC. Long-term outcomes after radiosurgery for acoustic neuromas. *N Engl J Med* 1998;339(20):1426-1433.

22 Fraass BA, Kessler ML, McShan DL, et al. Optimization and clinical use of multisegment intensity-modulated radiation therapy for high-dose conformal therapy. *Semin Radiat Oncol* 1999; 9(1):60-77.

23 Varlotto JM, Shrieve DC, Alexander E, et al. Fractionated stereotactic radiosurgery for the treatment of acoustic neuromas: preliminary results. *Int J Radiat Oncol Biol Phys* 1996; 36 (1):141-145.

24 Stehling L, Spence R, Contreras M, et al., editors. *Transfusion Medicine and Alternatives to Blood Transfusion.* Paris: R&J Éditions Médicales; 2000.

25 deAndrade JR. Prudent Strategies for Red Blood Cell Conservation in Orthopedic Surgery. *Am J Med* 1996;101(2A suppl): 16S-21S

26 Salem MR, Manley S. Blood conservation techniques. In: Salem MR, ed. *Blood Conservation in the Surgical Patient.* Baltimore: Williams & Wilkins; 1996:92-106.

27 Gombotz H, Metzler H, List WF. Methods for reduction of perioperative bleeding. *Br J Anaesth.* 1998;81(Suppl 1):62-66.

28 Czinn EA, Chediak JR. Coagulation and Hemostasis. In: Salem MR, ed. *Blood Conservation in the Surgical Patient.* Baltimore: Williams & Wilkins; 1996:45-78.

29 Thomas JM. Nonblood management in obstetrics and gynaecology. *J Soc Obstet Gynaecol Can* 1997;19(5):475-8.

30 Erber WN. The Haematology of Bloodless Surgery. *Bloodless Surgery Update* 1997;2(1):1-2

31 Nelson CL, Fontenot HJ. Ten Strategies to Reduce Blood Loss in Orthopedic Surgery. *Am J Surg* 1995;170(suppl 6A):64S-68S.

32 Despotis GJ, Joist JH, Hogue CW, Alsoufiev A, Kater K, Goodnough LT, et al. Individualized patient heparinization and protamine reversal. *J Thorac Cardiovasc Surg* 1996;111(2):493-494.

33 Despotis GJ, Joist JH, Goodnough LT. Monitoring of hemostasis in cardiac surgical patients: impact of point-of-care testing on blood loss and transfusion outcomes. *Clin Chem* 1997;43(9):1684-1696.

34 ViÒuela F, Canalis RF, Hartz RS, et al. Surgical hemostasis and blood conservation. In: Salem MR, ed. *Blood Conservation in the Surgical Patient.* Baltimore: Williams & Wilkins; 1996:386-424.

35 Ishiwata Y, Inomori S, Fujitsu K, et al. A new intracranial silastic encircling clip for hemostasis. *J Neurosurg* 1990;73(4):638-639.

36 Patsner B, Orr JW. Intractable venous sacral hemorrhage: Use of stainless steel thumbtacks to obtain hemostasis. *Am J Obs Gyn* 1990;162(2):452.

37 DeAndrade JR. Prudent Strategies for Red Blood Cell Conservation in Orthopedic Surgery. *Am J Med* 1996;101(suppl 2A):16S-21S.

38 Salem MR, Manley S. Blood conservation techniques. In: Salem MR, ed. *Blood Conservation in the Surgical Patient.* Baltimore: Williams & Wilkins; 1996:92-106.

39 Achauer BM, Hernandez J, Parker A. Burn Excision with Intraoperative Vasopressin. *J Burn Care Rehab* 1989;10:375-378

40 Appleton DS, Sibley GN, Doyle PT. Internal iliac artery embolisation for the control of severe bladder and prostate haemorrhage. *Br J Urol* 1988;61(1):45-7.

41 Collins CD, Jackson JE. Pelvic arterial embolization following hysterectomy and bilateral internal iliac artery ligation for intractable primary postpartum haemorrhage. *Clin Radiol* 1995; 50:710-714.

42 Pelage JP, Soyer P, Repiquet D, et al. Secondary postpartum hemorrhage: treatment with selective arterial embolization. *Radiology* 1999; 212(2):385-9

43 Kubba AK, Palmer KR. Role of endoscopic injection therapy in the treatment of bleeding peptic ulcer. *Br J Surg* 1996;83(4):461-468.

44 Leu HF, Hauser RK. Percutaneous endoscopic lumbar spine fusion. *Neurosurg Clin N Am* 1996;7(1):107-117.

45 Fann JI, Pompili MF, Stevens JH, et al. Port-access cardiac operations with cardioplegic arrest. *Ann Thorac Surg* 1997;63(suppl 6):S35-S39.

46 Lam D, Miranda R, Hom SJ. Laparoscopic cholecystectomy as an outpatient procedure. *J Am Coll Surg* 1997;185(2):152-155.

47 Coombs R, Hughes B, Zhou SH. How Can the Surgeon Limit Perioperative Bleeding? The Example of Orthopaedic Surgery. In: Belghiti J, Castot M, Conseiller C, et al., eds. *Bloodless Surgery: Surgical and Anaesthetic Aspects; Legal and Ethical Issues.* Paris: Arnette Blackwell; 1997:15-8.

48 Brodsky JW, Dickson JH, Erwin WD, et al. Hypotensive anesthesia for scoliosis surgery in Jehovah's Witnesses. *Spine* 1991;16(3):304-6.

49 Nelson CL, Fontenot HJ. Ten Strategies to Reduce Blood Loss in Orthopedic Surgery. *Am J Surg* 1995;170(suppl 6A):64S-68S.

50 Salem MR, Manley S. Blood Conservation Techniques. In: Salem MR, ed. *Blood Conservation in the Surgical Patient.* Baltimore: Williams & Wilkins; 1996:92-106.

51 Milani JC. Blood preservation in spine surgery: an overview. *Spine: State Art Rev* 1991;5(1):17-27.

52 Murphy JM. Anesthetic considerations in lumbar spinal surgery. *Spine: State Art Rev* 1991;5(1):29-33.

53 Bragg LE, Thompson JS. Management strategies in the Jehovah's Witness patient. *Contemp Surg* 1990;36:45-9.

54 deAndrade JR. Prudent Strategies for Red Blood Cell Conservation in Orthopedic Surgery. *Am J Med* 1996;101(2A suppl): 16S-21S

55 Salem MR, Manley S. Blood conservation techniques. In: Salem MR, ed. *Blood Conservation in the Surgical Patient.* Baltimore: Williams & Wilkins; 1996: 92-106.

56 Nelson CL, Bowen WS. Total Hip Arthroplasty in Jehovah's Witnesses without Blood Transfusion. *J Bone and Joint Surg* 1986;68-A(3):350-353

57 Petrozza PH. Induced hypotension. *Int Anesthiol Clin* 1990;28(4):223-9.

58 Stein JI, Gombotz H, Rigler B, et al. Open Heart Surgery in Children of Jehovah's Witnesses: Extreme Hemodilution on Cardiopulmonary Bypass. *Pediatr Cardiol* 1991;12:170-174

59 Crystal GJ, Salem MR, Acute Normovolemic Hemodilution. In: Salem MR, editor. *Blood Conservation in the Surgical Patient.* Baltimore: Williams & Wilkins; 1996:168-188.

60 Schmied H, Kurz A, Sessler DI, et al. Mild hypothermia increases blood loss and transfusion requirements during total hip arthroplasty. *Lancet* 1996;347(8997):289-292.

61 Bush HL, Hydo LJ, Fischer E, et al. Hypothermia during elective abdominal aortic aneurysm repair: the high price of avoidable morbidity. *J Vasc Surg* 1995;21(1):392-402.

62 Tawes RL Jr., ed. *Autotransfusion: Therapeutic Principles and Trends.* Detroit: Gregory Appleton; 1997.

63 Spence RK. Blood Management Practice Guidelines Conference. Surgical red blood cell transfusion practice policies. *Am J Surg* 1995:170(suppl 6A):3S-15S.

64 Schaller RT, Schaller J, Morgan A, Furman EB. Hemodilution Anesthesia: A Valuable Aid to Major Cancer Surgery in Children. *Am J Surg* 1983;146:79-84

65 Grubbs PE Jr., Marini CP, Fleischer A. Acute hemodilution in an anemic Jehovah's Witness during extensive abdominal wall resection and reconstruction. *Ann Plast Surg* 1989;22(5):448-52.

66 Kafer ER, Collins ML. Acute intraoperative hemodilution and perioperative blood salvage. *Anesth Clin North Am* 1990;8(3):543-67.

67 Monk TG, Goodnough LT. Blood Conservation Strategies to Minimize Allogeneic Blood Use in Urologic Surgery. *Am.J Surg* 1995;170(6A suppl):69S-73S

68 Goodnough LT. Acute Normovolemic Hemodilution. *Transfusion Alternatives in Transfusion Medicine* 1999;1(1):12-16.

69 Monk TG, Goodnough LT. Acute Normovolemic Hemodilution. *Clinical Orthopaedics and Related Research* 1998;357:74-81.

70 Monk TG, Goodnough LT, Brecher ME, et al. A Prospective Randomized Comparison of Three Blood Conservation Strategies for Radical Prostatectomy. *Anesthesiology* 1999;91(1):24-33.

71 Trouwborst A, van Woerkens ECSM, van Daele M, Tenbrinck R. Acute hypervolaemic haemodilution to avoid blood transfusion during major surgery. *Lancet* 1990; 336(8726):1295-7.

72 Trouwborst A, Hagenouw RRPM, Jeekel J, Ong GL. Hypervolaemic haemodilution in an anaemic Jehovah's Witness. *Brit J Anaesth* 1990;64(5):646-8.

73 Stehling L. Autologous transfusion. *Int Anesthesiol Clin* 1990 Fall;28(4):190-6.

74 Consensus Statement: Autologous transfusion – 3 years on: What is new? *Transfusion Medicine* 1999;9:285-286.

75 Royal College of Physicians of Edinburgh Consensus Conference on Autologous Transfusion November 1998. Desmond M, Gillon J, Thomas MJG. Perioperative red cell salvage: a case for implementing the 1995 consensus statement. *Transfusion Medicine* 1999;9:265-268.

76 Joseph NJ, Kamaryt J, Paulissian R. Blood Salvage Techniques. In: Salem MR, ed. *Blood Conservation in the Surgical Patient.* Williams & Wilkins; 1996:252-304.

77 Thomas MJG. Infected and malignant fields are an absolute contraindication to intraoperative cell salvage: fact or fiction? Royal College of Physicians of Edinburgh Consensus Conference on Autologous Transfusion November 1998. *Transfusion Medicine* 1999;9:269-278.

78 Edelman MJ, Potter P, Mahaffey KG, et al. The potential for reintroduction of tumor cells during intraoperative blood salvage: reduction of risk with use of the RC-400 leukocyte depletion filter. *Urology* 1996;47(2):179-181.

79 Stehling L, Zauder HL, Vertrees R. Alternatives to allogeneic transfusion. In: Petz LD, Swisher SN, Kleinman S, et al, editors. *Clinical Practice of Transfusion Medicine,* (3rd ed). New York: Churchill Livingstone; 1996: 539-561.

80 Christensen JT, Reuse J, Badel P, et al. Plateletpheresis before redo CABG diminishes excessive blood transfusion. *Ann Thorac Surg* 1996;62:1373-9.

81 Ramos HC, Todo S, Kang Y, Felekouras E, Doyle H, Starzl TE. Liver Transplantation Without the Use of Blood Products. *Arch Surg* 1994;129:528-33.

82 Potter PS. Utilization of Autologous Transfusion Technologies for Allogeneic-blood-free Cardiac Transplantation in Pediatric Patients. *Transfusion Alternatives in Transfusion Medicine* 1999;1(1):26-28

83 Semkiw LB, Schurman DJ, Goodman SB, Woolson ST. Postoperative Blood Salvage Using the Cell Saver after Total Joint Arthroplasty. *J Bone and Joint* 1989;71-A(6):823-27.

84 Sculco TP. Blood Management in Orthopedic Surgery. *Am J Surg* 1995;170(suppl 1):60S-63S.

85 Rosengart TK, Helm RE, DeBois J, et al. Open heart operations without transfusion using a multimodality blood conservation strategy in 50 Jehovah's Witness patients: implications for a "bloodless" surgical technique. *J Am Coll Surg* 1997;184:618-629

86 Gurbuz AT, Novick WM, Pierce CA, Watson DC. Impact of ultrafiltration on blood use for atrial septal defect closure in infants and children. *Ann Thorac Surg* 1998;65(4):1105-1108.

87 Estioko MR, Litwak RS, Rand JH. Reoperation, Emergency and Urgent Open Cardiac Surgery in Jehovah's Witnesses. *Chest* 1992;102:50-53

88 Rousou JA, Engleman RM, Flack JE 3rd, et al. The 'primeless pump': a novel technique for intraoperative blood conservation. *Cardiovasc Surg* 1999;7(2):228-235.

89 Habler O, Mebmer K. Hyperoxaemia in extreme haemodilution. *Br J Anaesth* 1998;81(suppl 1):79-82.

90 Dupuis JF, Nguyen DT. Anesthetic Management of the Patient Who Refuses Blood Transfusions. *The Cancer Bulletin* 1995;47(1):67-73.

91 Spence RK, Cernaianu AC. Pharmacological Agents as Adjuncts to Bloodless Vascular Surgery. *Seminars in Vascular Surgery* 1994;7(2):114-120

92 Fremes SE, et al. Metaanalysis of Prophylactic Drug Treatment in the Prevention of Postoperative Bleeding. *Ann Thorac Surg* 1994;58:1580-88.

93 Chernow B. Blood Conservation - A Critical Care Imperative. *Crit Care Med* 1991;19(3):313-14

94 Smoller BR, Kruskall MS, Horowitz GL. Reducing adult phlebotomy blood loss with the use of pediatric-sized blood collection tubes. *Am J Clin Pathol* 1989;91(6):701-703.

95 Corwin HL, Parsonnet KC, Gettinger A. RBC transfusion in the ICU. Is there a reason? *Chest* 1995;108(3):767-771.

96 Mock T, Morrison D, Yatscoff R. Evaluation of the i-STAT system: a portable chemistry analyzer for the measurement of sodium, potassium, chloride, urea, glucose, and hematocrit. *Clin Biochem* 1995;28(2):187-92.

97 Civetta JM, Hudson-Civetta JA. Maintaining quality of care while reducing charges in the ICU. Ten ways. *Ann Surg* 1985;202(4):524-532.

98 Griffel MI, Kaufman BS. Pharmacology of Colloids and Crystalloids. *Critical Care Clinics* 1992;8(2):235-253.

99 Haljamäe H. Use of fluids in trauma. *International Journal of Intensive Care* 1999:20-29.

100 Boldt J. Choice of a Synthetic Colloid for Surgery. *Transfusion Alternatives in Transfusion Medicine* 1999;1(1):18-25.

101 Elliott R, Fluid replacement strategies. In: Elliot R, ed. *Critical Care Therapeutics*. London: Pharmaceutical Press;1999:97-103.

102 McEvoy GK, Welsh OH, Snow EK, et al., eds. *AHFS Drug Information*. Bethesda, MD: American Society of Health-System Pharmacists;1999.

103 Dextran 1. In: Parfitt K, ed. Martindale: The complete drug reference, 32nd ed. London: Pharmaceutical Press;1999.

104 Royston D. Blood-sparing drugs: aprotinin, tranexamic acid, and epsilon-aminocaproic acid. *Int Anesthesiol Clin.* 1995; Winter;33(1):155-79.

105 Spence RK, Cernaianu AC. Pharmacological agents as adjuncts to bloodless vascular surgery. *Semin Vasc Surg* 1994;7(2):114-120.

106 Chen RH, Frazier OH, Cooley DA. Antifibrinolytic therapy in cardiac surgery. *Tex Heart Inst J* 1995;22(3):211-5.

107 Garewal H, Durie BGM. Anti-fibrinolytic therapy with aminocaproic acid for the control of bleeding in thrombocytopenic patients. *Scand J Haematol* 1985; 35:497-500.

108 Bartholomew JR, Salgia R, Bell WR. Control of Bleeding in Patients With Immune and Nonimmune Thrombocytopenia With Aminocaproic Acid. *Arch Intern Med* 1989;149:1959-1961.

109 Karski JM, Teasdale SJ, Norman P, et al. Prevention of bleeding after cardiopulmonary bypass with high-dose tranexamic acid. *J Thorac Cardiovasc Surg* 1995;110(3):835-42.

110 Dryden PJ, O'Connor JP, Jamieson WR, et al. Tranexamic acid reduces blood loss and transfusion in reoperative cardiac surgery. *Can J Anaesth* 1997;44(9):934-941.

111 Boylan JF, Klinck JR, Sandler AN, et al. Tranexamic acid reduces blood loss, transfusion requirements, and coagulation factor use in primary orthotopic liver transplantation. *Anesthesiol* 1996;85(5):1043-1048.

112 Hiippala ST, Strid LJ, Wennerstrand MI, et al. Tranexamic acid radically decreases blood loss and transfusion associated with total knee arthroplasty. *Anesth Analg* 1997;84(4):839-844.

113 Benoni G. Tranexamic acid reduces the blood loss in knee arthroplasty – if it's administered at the right time. *Lakartidningen* 1999;96(24):2967-2969.

114 Patrassi GM, Viero M, Sartori MT, et al. Aprotinin efficacy on intraoperative bleeding and transfusion requirements in orthotopic liver transplantation. *Transfusion* 1994;34:507-511

115 Cicek S, Demirkilic U, Kuralay E, et al. Postoperative aprotinin: effect on blood loss and transfusion requirements in cardiac operations. *Ann Thorac Surg* 1996;61(5):1372-6.

116 Taylor KM. Aprotinin therapy and blood conservation: extending the indications. *Br J Surg* 1992;79(12):1258-9.

117 Murkin JM, Shannon NA, Bourne RB, et al. Aprotinin decreases blood loss in patients undergoing revision or bilateral total hip arthroplasty. *Anesth Analg* 1995;80(2):343-48.

118 Capdevila X, Calvet Y, Biboulet P, et al. Aprotinin decreases blood loss and homologous transfusions in patients undergoing major orthopedic surgery. *Anesthesiology* 1998;88(1):50-57.

119 Seu P, Neelankanta G, Csete M, et al. Liver transplantation for fulminant hepatic failure in a Jehovah's Witness. *Clin Transplant* 1996;10(5):404-407

120 Kobrinsky NL, Tulloch H. Treatment of refractory thrombocytopenic bleeding with 1-desamino-8-d-arginine vasopressin (desmopressin). *J Pediatr* 1988;112(6):993-6.

121 Douglas JT, Shaw J. High-dose desmopressin in bleeding disorders. *Eur J Anaesthesiol* 1997;14(Suppl 14):v-vi.

122 Achauer BM, Hernandez J, Parker A. Burn excision with intraoperative vasopressin. *J Burn Care Rehab* 1989;10(4):375-8.

123 Fletcher H, Frederick J, Hardie M, Simeon D. A randomized comparison of vasopressin and tourniquet as hemostatic agents during myomectomy. *Obstet Gynecol* 1996;87(6):1014-1018.

124 Mosconi G, Mambelli E, Zanchelli F, et al. Severe gastrointestinal bleeding in a uremic patient treated with estrogen-progesterone therapy. *Int J Artif Organs* 1999;22(5):313-316.

125 Tran A, Villeneuve JP, Bilodeau M, et al. Treatment of chronic bleeding from gastric antral vascular ectasia (GRAVE) with estrogen-progesterone in cirrhotic patients: an open pilot study. *Am J Gastroenterol* 1999;94(10):2909-2911.

126 Barkin JS, Ross BS. Medical therapy for chronic gastrointestinal bleeding of obscure origin. *Am J Gastroenterol* 1998;93(8):1250-1254.

127 Leach M, Makris M, Hampton KK, Preston FE. Norethisterone therapy for bleeding due to gastrointestinal telangiectases in Glanzmann's thrombasthenia. *Br J Haematol* 1998;100(3):594-596.

128 Chuong CJ, Brenner PF. Management of abnormal uterine bleeding. *Am J Obstet Gynecol* 1996;175(3 Pt 2):787-792.

129 Alparin JB. Letter. *Transf Med Rev* 1995;IX(4):339

130 Czinn EA, Chediak JR. Coagulation and Hemostasis. In: Salem MR, ed. *Blood Conservation in the Surgical Patient.* Baltimore: Williams & Wilkins; 1996:45-78

131 Kram HB, Evans T, Clark SR, et al. Techniques of hepatic hemostasis using fibrin glue. *Contemp Surg* 1990;37(3):11-15.

132 Kram HB, Ragu CN, Stafford FJ, et al. Fibrin glue achieves hemostasis in patients with coagulation disorders. *Arch Surg* 1989;124:385-387.

133 Gombotz H, Metzler H, List WF. Methods for reduction of perioperative bleeding. *Br J Anaesth* 1998;81(suppl 1):62-66.

134 Bachet J, Goudot B, Dreyfus G, et al. The proper use of glue: a 20-year experience with the GRF glue in acute aortic dissection. *Journal of Cardiovascular Surgery* 1997;12 (suppl 2):243-253.

135 Levy O, Martinowitz U, Oran A, et al. The use of fibrin tissue adhesive to reduce blood loss and the need for blood transfusion after total knee arthroplasty. A prospective, randomized, multicenter study. *J Bone Joint Surg Am* 1999;81(11):1580-1588.

136 Tawes RL, Sydorak GR, DuVall TB. Autologous fibrin glue: the last step in operative hemostasis. *Am J Surg* 1994;168(2):120-122.

137 Gibble JW, Ness PM. Current Perspectives on the Use of Fibrin Glue (Sealant) in the United States in the 1990s. In: Tawes RL Jr., ed. *Autotransfusion: Therapeutic Principles and Trends.* Detroit: Gregory Appleton;1997:250-259.

138 Whitman DH, Berry RL, Gree DM. Platelet gel: an autologous alternative to fibrin glue with applications in oral and maxillofacial surgery. *J Oral Maxillofac Surg* 1997;55(11):1294-1299.

139 Thomas JM, Wong CJ, Bodnaruk ZM, et al. Clinical Strategies for Managing Hemorrhage and Anemia Without Blood Transfusion in the ICU. *ICU 97 Abstract No. 726.* ON: Canada; 1997.

140 Dudrick SJ, O'Donnell JJ, Raleigh DP, et al. Rapid restoration of red blood cell mass in severely anemic surgical patients who refuse transfusion. *Arch Surg* 1985;120:721-7.

141 Horl WH, Cavill I, MacDougall IC, et al. How to diagnose and correct iron deficiency during r-huEPO therapy - a consensus report. *Nephrol Dial Transplant* 1996;11:246-250

142 Swain RA, Kaplan B, Montgomery E. Iron deficiency anemia. When is parenteral therapy warranted? *Postgrad Med* 1996;100(5):181-92.

143 Monaghan MS, Glasco G, St. John G, et al. Safe administration of iron dextran to a patient who reacted to the test dose. *South Med J* 1994;87:1010-1012.

144 Breymann C, Zimmerman R, Huch R, et al. Use of recombinant human erythropoietin in combination with parenteral iron in the treatment of postpartum anaemia. *Eur J Clin Invest* 1996;26(2):123-130.

[145] Hallberg L, Brune M, Rossander-Hulthen L. Is there a physiological role of vitamin C in iron absorption? *Ann N Y Acad Sci* 1987;498:324-32.

[146] Estioko MR, Litwak RS, Rand JH. Reoperation, Emergency and Urgent Open Cardiac Surgery in Jehovah's Witnesses. *Chest* 1992;102:50-53

[147] Atabek U, Alvarez R, Pello MJ, et al. Erythropoietin accelerates hematocrit recovery in post-surgical anemia. *Am Surg* 1995;61(1):74-7.

[148] Goodnough LT, Monk TG, Andriole GL. Erythropoietin therapy. *N Engl J Med* 1997;336(13):933-8.

[149] Koestner JA, Nelson LD, Morris JA Jr., et al. Use of recombinant human erythropoietin (r-HuEPO) in a Jehovah's Witness refusing transfusion of blood products. *J Trauma* 1990;30(11):1406-8.

[150] Kraus P, Lipman J. Erythropoietin in a patient following multiple trauma. *Anaesth* 1992;47(11):962-4.

[151] Rutherford CJ, Schneider TJ, Dempsey H, et al. Efficacy of different dosing regimens for recombinant human erythropoietin in a simulated perisurgical setting: the importance of iron availability in optimizing response. *Am J Med* 1994;96(2):139-45.

[152] Wolff M, Fandrey J, Hirner A, et al. Perioperative use of recombinant human erythropoietin in patients refusing blood transfusions. Pathophysiological considerations based on 5 cases. *Eu J Haematol* 1997;58:154-159.

[153] Van Wyck DB. Iron management during recombinant human erythropoietin therapy. *Am J Kidney Dis* 1989;XIV(2 suppl 1):9-13.

[154] Faris PM, Ritter MA, Abels RI, et al. The effects of recombinant human erythropoietin on perioperative transfusion requirements in patients having a major orthopaedic operation. *J Bone Joint Surg* 1996;78A(1):62-72.

[155] Porter JC, Leahey A, Polise K, et al. Recombinant human erythropoietin reduces the need for erythrocyte and platelet transfusions in pediatric patients with sarcoma: a randomized double-blind, placebo-controlled trial. *J Pediatr* 1996;129(5):656-660.

[156] Cazzola M, Mercuriali F, Brungnara C. Use of Recombinant Human Erythropoietin Outside the Setting of Uremia. *Blood* 1997;89(12):4248-4246.

[157] Corwin HL, Gettinger A, Rodriguez RM, et al. Efficacy of recombinant human erythropoietin in the critically ill patient: a randomized, double-blind, placebo-controlled trial. *Crit Care Med* 1999;27(11):2346-2350.

[158] Pronai W, Riegler-Keil M, Silberbauer K, et al. Folic acid supplementation improves erythropoietin response. *Nephron* 1995;71(4):395-400.

[159] Green R. Screening for vitamin B12 deficiency: caveat emptor. *Ann Intern Med* 1996;124(5):509-511.

[160] Ballal SH, Domoto DT, Polack DC, et al. Androgens potentiate the effects of erythropoietin in the treatment of anemia of end-stage renal disease. *Am J Kidney Dis* 1991;17(1):29-33.

[161] Teruel JL, Marcen R, Navarro-Antolin J, et al. Androgen versus erythropoietin for the treatment of anemia in hemodialyzed patients: a prospective study. *J Am Soc Nephrol* 19967(1):140-144.

[162] Dudrick SJ, O'Donnell JJ, Raleigh DP, et al. Rapid restoration of red blood cell mass in severely anemic surgical patients who refuse transfusion. *Arch Surg* 1985;120:721-7.

[163] Brimacombe J, Skippen P, Talbutt P. Acute anaemia to a haemoglobin of 14 g.l⁻¹ with survival. *Anaesth Intens Care* 1991;19(4):581-3.

[164] Mann MC, Votto J, Kambe J, McNamee MJ. Management of the Severely Anemic Patient Who Refuses Transfusion: Lessons Learned during the Care of a Jehovah's Witness. *Ann Intern Med* 1992;117(12):1042-1048.

[165] Bickell WH, Shaftan GW, Mattox KL. Intravenous fluid administration and uncontrolled hemorrhage. *J Trauma* 1989;29(3):409.

[166] Shoemaker WC, Peitzman AB, Bellamy R, et al. Resuscitation from severe hemorrhage. *Crit Care Med* 1996;24(2 Suppl.):S12-23.

[167] Stehling L, Zauder HL. How low can we go? Is there a way to know? *Transfusion* 1990; 30(1):1-3.

[168] Howell PJ, Bamber PA. Severe acute anemia in a Jehovah's Witness. *Anaesth* 1987;42(1):44-8.

162

[169] Kraus P, Lipman J. Erythropoietin in a patient following multiple trauma. *Anaesth* 1992;47(11):962-4.

[170] Kikura M. Levy JH. New cardiac drugs. *Int Anesthesiol Clin* 1995;33(1):21-37.

[171] Levy B, Bollaert PE, Bauer P, et al. Therapeutic optimization including inhaled nitric oxide in adult respiratory distress syndrome in a polyvalent intensive care unit. *J Trauma* 1995;38(3):370-374.

[172] Third European Consensus Conference in Intensive Care Medicine. Tissue hypoxia: How to detect, how to correct, how to prevent. Societe de Reanimation de Langue Francaise. The American Thoracic Society. European Society of Intensive Care Medicine. *Am J Respir Crit Care Med* 1996;154(5):1573-8

[173] Fischer B, Jain KK, Braun E, et al. Effect of Hyperbaric Oxygenation on Disorders of the Blood: Hypovolemia and Acute Anemia Due to Blood Loss. *Handbook of Hyperbaric Oxygen Therapy.* Berlin: Springer-Verlag; 1988:180-3.

[174] Grim PS, Gottlieb LJ, Boddie A, et al. Hyperbaric Oxygen Therapy. *JAMA* 1990;263(16):2216-20.

[175] Tibbles PM, Edelsberg JS. Hyperbaric Oxygen Therapy. *N Engl J Med* 1996;334(25):1642-48.

[176] Stehling L, Zauder HL. How low can we go? Is there a way to know? *Transfusion* 1990;30(1):1-3.

[177] Greenwalt TJ, Buckwalter JA, Desforger J, et al. Consensus conference. Perioperative red blood cell transfusion. *JAMA* 1988;260(18):2700-3.

[178] Dietrich KA, Conrad SA, Hebert CA, Levy GL, Romero MD. Cardiovascular and metabolic response to red blood cell transfusion in critically ill volume-resuscitated nonsurgical patients. *Crit Care Med* 1990;18(9):940-4.

[179] Spence RK. Emerging Trends in Surgical Blood Transfusion. *Seminars in Hematology* 1997;34(3):48-53.

[180] Welch HG, Meehan KR, Goodnough LT. Prudent Strategies for Elective Red Blood Cell Transfusion. *Ann Intern Med* 1992;116(5):393-402.

[181] American College of Physicians. Clinical Guidelines: Practice Strategies for Elective Red Blood Cell Transfusions. *Ann Intern Med* 1992;116(5):404-406.

[182] Chen AY, Carson JL. Perioperative management of anemia. *Br J Anaesth* 1998;81(suppl 1):20-24

[183] Spence RK. Preoperative packed cell volume necessary for patients undergoing elective surgery. *Br J Anaesth* 1998;81(suppl 1):50-55.

[184] Hebert PC, Wells G, Blajchman MA, et al. A Multicenter, Randomized, Controlled Clinical Trial of Transfusion Requirements in Critical Care. *N Engl J Med* 1999;340:409-417.

[185] Bracey AW, Radovancevic R, Riggs SA, et al. Lowering the hemoglobin threshold for transfusion in coronary artery bypass procedures: effect on patient outcome. *Transfusion* 1999;39(10):1070-1077.

[186] Akingbola OA, Custer JR, Bunchman TE, Sedman AB. Management of severe anemia without transfusion in a pediatric Jehovah's Witness patient. *Critical Care Medicine* 1994;22(3):524-28.

[187] Nearman HS, Eckhauser ML. Postoperative management of a severely anemic Jehovah's Witness. *Crit Care Med* 1983;11(2):142-3.

[188] Vadhan-Raj S. Recombinant human erythropoietin in combination with other hematopoietic cytokines in attenuating chemotherapy-induced multilineage myelosuppression: brief communication. *Semin Hematol* 1996;18(suppl 1):16-18.

[189] Bessho M, Hirashima K, Asano S, et al. Multicenter Study Group. Treatment of the anemia of aplastic anemia patients with recombinant human erythropoietin in combination with granulocyte colony-stimulating factor: a multicenter randomized controlled study. *Eur J Haematol* 1997;58(4):265-272.

[190] Lifton R, Bennett JM. Clinical use of granulocyte-macrophage colony-stimulating factor and granulocyte colony-stimulating factor in neutropenia associated with malignancy. *Hematol Oncol Clin N Am* 1996;10(4):825-839.

[191] Du X, Williams DA. Interleukin-11: review of molecular, cell biology, and clinical use. *Blood* 1997;89(11):3897-3908.

192 Tepler I, Elias L, Smith JW, et al. A randomized placebo-controlled trial of recombinant human interleukin-11 in cancer patients with severe thrombocytopenia due to chemotherapy. *Blood* 1996;87(9):3607-3614.

193 Isaacs C, Robert NJ, Bailey FA, et al. Randomized placebo-controlled study of recombinant human interleukin-11 to prevent chemotherapy-induced thrombocytopenia in patients with breast cancer receiving dose-intensive cyclophosphamide and doxorubicin. *J Clin Oncol* 1997;15:3368-3377.

194 Vadhan-Raj S, Murray LJ, Bueso-Ramos C. Stimulation of megakaryocyte and platelet production by a single dose of recombinant human thrombopoietin in patients with cancer. *Ann Intern Med* 1997;126(9):673-681.

195 Somlo G, Sniecinski I, ter Veer A, et al. Recombinant human thrombopoietin in combination with granulocyte colony-stimulating factor enhances mobilization of peripheral blood progenitor cells, increases peripheral blood platelet concentration, and accelerates hematopoietic recovery following high-dose chemotherapy. *Blood* 1999;93(9):2798-2806.

196 Wu HK, Chiba S, Hirai H, et al. Effect of stem cell factor (c-kit Ligand) on clonogenic leukemic precursor cells: synergy with other hematopoietic growth factors. *Am J Hematol* 1994;47(4):328-330.

197 Gould SA. Sehgal LR, Sehgal HL, Moss GS. Blood Substitutes. In: Salem MR, ed. *Blood Conservation in the Surgical Patient*. Baltimore: Williams & Wilkins; 1996: 92-106.

198 Baron JF. Haemoglobin therapy in clinical practice: use and characteristics of DCLb. *Br J Anaesth* 1998;81(suppl 1):34-37.

199 Spahn DR. van Brempt R, Theilmeier G, et al. Perflubron emulsion delays blood transfusions in orthopedic surgery. European Perflubron Emulsion Study Group. *Anesthesiology* 1999;91(5):1195-1208.

200 Spahn DR. Blood Substitutes. Artificial oxygen carriers: Perfluorocarbon emulsions. *Critical Care* 1999; 3(5): R93-R97.

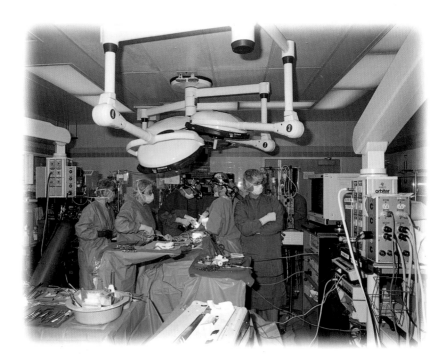

APPENDIX 3

BLOODLESS SURGERY CENTERS WORLDWIDE

United States of America

- Allegheny General Hospital - Pittsburgh, PA
- Alvarado Hospital Medical Center - San Diego, CA
- Anaheim General Hospital Information Services - Anaheim, CA
- Bridgeport Hospital - Bridgeport, CT
- Brookdale University Hospital Medical Center - Brooklyn, NY
- Brookwood Medical Center - Birmingham, AL
- Brotman Medical Center - Culver City, CA
- Buffalo General Hospital - Buffalo, NY
- Center for Bloodless Medicine and Surgery – Graduate Hospital - Philadelphia, PA
- Centinela Hospital Medical Center - Inglewood, CA
- Coast Plaza Doctor's Hospital - Norwalk, CA
- Community Hospital of Los Gatos - Los Gatos, CA
- Community Memorial Hospital - Ventura, CA
- Cooper Hospital-University Medical Center - Camden, NJ, US
- Coral Gables Hospital - Coral Gables, FL
- Corona Regional Medical Center - Corona, CA
- DCH Regional Medical Center - Tuscaloosa, AL
- Desert Regional Medical Center - Palms Springs, CA
- Doctor's Medical Center - Modesto, CA
- Encino-Tarzana Regional Medical Center - Tarzana, CA
- Florida Medical Center - Fort Lauderdale, FL
- Flower Hospital - Sylvania, OH
- Fountain Valley Regional Hospital and Medical Center - Fountain Valley, CA
- French Hospital and Medical Center - San Luis, Obispo, CA
- Genesys Regional Medical Center - Grand Blanc, MI
- Glendale Memorial Hospital and Health Center - Glendale, CA
- Good Samaritan Hospital - Bakersfield, CA
- Good Samaritan Hospital - Los Angeles, CA
- Good Samaritan Regional Medical Center - Phoenix, AZ
- Gulf Coast Medical Center - Biloxi, MS
- Hackensack University Medical Center - Hackensack, NJ

- Hartford Hospital - Hartford, CT
- Hennepin County Medical Center - Minneapolis, MN
- Illinois Center for Bloodless Medicine and Surgery at Proctor Hospital - Peoria, IL
- John F. Kennedy Memorial Hospital - Indio, CA
- John Muir Medical Center - Walnut Creek, CA
- Kadlec Medical Center - Richland, WA
- Lake Mead Hospital Medical Center - N. Las Vegas, NV
- Legacy Portland Hospitals Good Samaritan and Emanuel Children's - Portland, OR
- Long Beach Community Medical Center - Long Beach, CA
- McKay-Dee Hospital Center - Ogden, UT
- Memorial Medical Center - New Orleans, LA
- Mercy Hospital - Detroit, MI
- Metropolitan Methodist Hospital - San Antonio, TX
- Mission Hospital - Mission, TX
- New York Methodist Hospital - Brooklyn, NY
- Northwest Community Hospital - Arlington Heights, IL
- Our Lady of the Resurrection Medical Center - Chicago, IL
- Palmetto General Hospital - Hialeah, FL
- Providence of Seattle Medical Center - Seattle, WA
- Puget Sound Hospital - Tacoma, WA
- Rhode Island Hospital - Providence, RI
- Roper Hospital - Charleston, SC
- Sahlgrenska University Hospital - Göteborg, SE
- Saint Clare Hospital - Tacoma, WA
- Saint Francis Hospital - Federal Way, WA
- Saint Joseph Hospital at Creighton University Medical Center - Omaha, NE
- Saint Joseph's Medical Center - Tacoma, WA
- San Ramon Regional Medical Center - San Ramon,CA
- Sierra Vista Regional Medical Center - San Luis Obispo, CA
- Sisters of Charity St. John Hospital - Nassau Bay, TX
- Sisters of Charity-St. Patrick Hospital - Lake Charles, LA
- St. Joseph's Hospital - Savannah, GA
- St. Jude Medical Center - Fullerton, CA
- St. Luke's Medical Center - Phoenix, AZ
- St. Luke's Medical Center - Pasadena, CA

- St. Mary's Health Services - Grand Rapids, MI
- St. Thomas Hospital - Nashville, TN
- St. Vincent Charity Hospital and Columbia St. John West Shore - Cleveland, OH
- St. Vincent's Hospital and Health Center - Billings, MT
- Staten Island University Hospital - Staten Island, NY
- Temple Community Hospital - Los Angeles, CA
- Tenet Doctors Hospital - Dallas, TX
- Tenet Park Place Med. Center & Mid Jefferson Hospital - Port Arthur, TX
- Tenet Park Plaza Hospital - Houston, TX
- The Center for Bloodless Medicine and Surgery, Pennsylvania Hospital - Philadelphia, PA
- The Cleveland Clinic Foundation - Cleveland, OH
- The Eugene and Mary B Meyer Center for Advanced Transfusion Practices, Johns Hopkins University School of Medicine, Baltimore, MD
- The New Jersey Institute for the Advancement of Bloodless Medicine and Surgery at Englewood Hospital and Medical Center - Englewood, NJ
- The New York Center for Bloodless Medicine and Surgery at the Long Island College Hospital - Brooklyn Heights, NY
- The New York Hospital-Cornell Medical Center - New York, NY
- The University Center for Bloodless Surgery and Medicine at UMDNJ-University Hospital - Newark, NJ
- Tri-City Regional Surgery Center - Richland, WA
- Trinity Medical Center - Carrollton, TX
- Tucson General Hospital - Tucson, AZ
- Tulsa Regional Medical Center - Tulsa, OK
- Twin Cities Community Hospital - Templeton, CA
- University Hospital - Denver, CO
- University Hospitals Health Systems, Rainbow Babies and Children's Hospital, Cleveland, OH
- University of Massachusetts Medical Center - Worcester, MA
- University of Miami - Jackson Memorial Hospital / Memorial Center - Miami, FL
- USC University Hospital - Los Angeles, CA
- USC Kenneth Norris Comprehensive Cancer Center and Hospital - Los Angeles, CA
- UT Bowld Hospital - Memphis, TN

- Valley Community Hospital - Santa Maria, CA
- Westchester Square Medical Center - Bronx, NY
- Western Medical Center Anaheim - Anaheim, CA
- Whittier Hospital Medical Center - Whittier, CA
- Winona Memorial Hospital - Indianapolis, IN

United Kingdom
- Ashtead Hospital, The Warren, Ashtead, Surrey KT21 2SB;
- Duchy Hospital, Preventinnie Lane, Treliske, Truro, Cornwall TR1 3UP;
- Fitzwilliam Hospital, Milton Way, South Bretton, Petersborough, Cambs PE3 9AQ;
- Mount Stuart Hospital, St Vincent's Road, Torquay, Devon TQ1 4UP;
- Oaks Hospital, 120 Mile End Road, Colchester, Essex CO4 5XR;
- Pinhill Hospital, Benslow Lane, Hitchin, Herts SG4 9QZ;
- The Rivers Hospital, Thomas Rivers Medical Centre, High Wych Road, Sawbridgeworth, Herts CM21 0HH;
- Springfield Medical Centre, Lawn Lane, Springfield, Chelmsford, Essex CM1 5GU;
- Winfield Hospital, Tewkesbury Road, Gloucester GL2 9EE;
- The Yorkshire Clinic, Bradford Road, Bingley, West Yorkshire BD16 1TW

Sweden
- Sahlgrenska University Hospital, Gothenburg;
- Lund University Hospital, Lund;
- Linkoping University Hospital, Linkoping;
- Nu-Medical Service, Uddevalla Hospital, Uddevalla

Israel
- Wolfson Medical Center

Australia
- Fremantle Kaleeya Hospital, East Fremantle 6158, WA

APPENDIX 4

GLOSSARY/WORDS TO RECOGNIZE

Initially, medical terms can be confusing and daunting to the lay reader. However, understanding the make-up of these words (their prefixes, suffixes and roots) can help demystify medical language. Following is a list of key words used in this book along with their components and basic meanings.

Acidosis [L. *acidus* sour + *osis* condition] a condition in which the blood pH is acidic.

Acute [L. *acutus* sharp] having a rapid onset and relatively short, severe course; as opposed to chronic.

AIDS acquired immunodeficiency syndrome.

Albumin [L. *albus* white + *in* in] a protein similar to that found in the white of egg (albumen). In blood, the major protein in plasma.

Allogeneic [Gr. *allos* other + *genein* to produce] tissues that are from the same species but antigenically or genetically different. Allogeneic blood is now the preferred term over homologous blood to define blood from another person for or in transfusion.

Anemia [Gr. *an* want or absence + *haima* blood + *ia* state or condition] lower than normal levels of red blood cells or their hemoglobin content.

Antibodies substances (immunoglobulins) produced by certain cells that interact with antigens to neutralize, inhibit or destroy them.

Anticoagulant [Gr. *anti* against + L. *coagulans* to drive together] any substance that prevents blood clotting.

Antifibrinolytic [Gr. *anti* against + L. *fibra* a fibre + Gr. *lysis* dissolution] inhibiting fibrinolysis. A substance that decreases fibrin breakdown.

Antigens [*antibody* + Gr. *gen* producing] any chemical substance that, under appropriate circumstances, causes the body to produce antibodies.

Arterial embolization see Embolization.

Autologous [Gr. *auto* self + *logos* relation] originating from self.

Autotransfusion [Gr. *auto* self + *transfusion*] the reinfusion of a patient's own blood or blood products. This can be done in one of four ways: 1. Collecting and storing the patient's blood before surgery for reinfusion at the time of surgery, 2. Withdrawal of the patient's blood or blood components in the operating room at the time of surgery for reinfusion at the conclusion of surgery, 3. Recycling the patient's blood collected from the operation site, or blood that has bled into a body cavity in trauma, and 4. Reinfusing blood collected from drains after surgery.

Bacteria [L.; Gr. *bakterion* little rod] Bacteria is the plural of bacterium. They are minute single-celled living microorganisms that multiply by cell division. Bacteria are classified in part by their shape. They are either spherical (coccal), rod-like (bacillary) or spiral/helical (spirochetal). They are further classified according to characteristics of their outer cell wall.

Blood count a determination of the number of blood cells (red blood cells, white blood cells and platelets) in a measured volume of blood, usually a cubic millimeter (mm3). These values can vary according to the test method used:

Red blood cell count:	Males	4.5 – 6.5 million/mm³
	Females	3.9 – 5.6 million/mm³
	Children	3.8 – 5.5 million/mm³ (varies according to age)
	Newborns	4.8 – 7.1 million/mm³
Hemoglobin:	Males	14 - 18 g/dL
	Females	12 - 16 g/dL
	Children	11 - 16 g/dL (varies according to age)
	Newborns	14 - 23 g/dL
Hematocrit:	Males	40% – 54%
	Females	38% - 47%
	Children	30% - 43% (varies according to age)
	Newborns	53% - 65%
White blood cell count – total:		5,000 - 10,000 /mm3
Platelet count:		150,000 - 400,000 /mm3.

Blood groups Blood grouping is a system of classifying the various blood types. They are determined by the presence of naturally occurring inherited antigens on the surface of blood cells. Approximately 400 red blood cell group antigens have been discovered. The best known and most clinically significant are the ABO and rhesus (Rh) group systems. The ABO grouping divides blood into four types: A, B, AB, and O. The rhesus system further divides each of the ABO blood types into either Rh-positive (Rh⁺) or Rh-negative (Rh⁻). Those with Rh antigens on their surface are classified as Rh⁺, and those without the Rh antigen as Rh⁻. There are also antigens on the surface of white blood cells, platelets and in plasma.

Intraoperative blood salvage (also **intraoperative cell salvage**) a procedure that uses a range of available devices to suction blood from the operating field. The machines then filter and return either whole blood or washed red blood cells to the patient.

Cardiac [Gr. *kardia* heart] pertaining to the heart; cardiac surgery.

Chronic [Gr. *chronos* time] a prolonged or long-term condition, as apposed to acute.

Citrate a form of citric acid used as an anticoagulant.

Coagulation [L. *co* together + *agere* to drive] the process of forming a clot.

Coagulation cascade [*coagulation* + cascade L. *cadere* to fall] the series of steps whereby the multiple coagulation factors are triggered and interact with each other to ultimately form a blood clot.

Coagulation factors substances (proteins) dissolved in the plasma that are an essential part of the clotting process. They are designated by Roman numerals, viz. Factor I = fibrinogen, Factor II = prothrombin, Factor III = thromboplastin, etc.

Coagulopathy any disorder of the blood clotting process.

Colloids [Gr. *kolla* glue + *eidos* form] A group of intravenous fluids used as volume expanders that contain small particles of proteins or other material such as starch or gelatin mixed but not dissolved in water. The size of the particles in colloids mean they do not readily pass through the capillary membrane and so remain mostly in the vascular compartment.

Component [L. *componere* to put together] the individual parts or elements making up a whole, e.g. the components of blood.

Component sequestration the therapeutic process of collecting blood from a patient at the time of surgery and separating out specific components, platelets, plasma and red cells, for later reinfusion.

Crystalloids [Gr. *krystallos* ice + *eidos* form] A group of intravenous fluids used as volume expanders which are a solution of salts and/or sugars dissolved in water. Crystalloid solutions freely pass through the capillary membrane.

Disease [Fr. *des* from + *aise* ease] Literally absence of ease and so any deviation from or disturbance of normal function or structure of a body part, organ or system, manifested by a set of signs or symptoms.

Edema [Gr. *oidema* swelling] the presence or accumulation of excessive fluid in the tissue spaces of the body.

Electrolytes [Gr. *elektron* amber (by rubbing amber an electric charge can be produced) + *lytos* soluble] Some compounds separate into chemically charged particles when dissolved in water. Collectively these dissolved charged particles are called electrolytes. To function properly, the body must maintain the correct concentration of electrolytes in the body's three fluid compartments. They serve three basic functions in the body: 1. Many are essential minerals, 2. They help control movement of water between body compartments, and 3. They help maintain the acid-base balance necessary for normal cellular activity.

Embolization [Gr. *embolos* plug] the therapeutic introduction of a substance into a blood vessel in order to obstruct or close off blood flow.

Enzymes [Gr. *en* in + *zyme* leaven] Substances that serve as catalysts which speed up chemical reactions.

Epoetin alfa recombinant human erythropoietin

Erythrocyte [Gr. *erythro* red + *kytos* cell] red blood cell.

Erythropoiesis [Gr. *erythro* red + *poiesis* making] the production of red blood cells.

Erythropoietin [Gr. *erythro* red + *poietes* maker] a hormone produced mainly in the kidneys of an adult which when released acts on stem cells in the bone marrow and stimulates the production of red blood cells. The synthetically produced product is referred to as recombinant human erythropoietin (r-HuEPO) or epoetin alfa.

et al. [L.] abbreviation for "and others."

Factor VIII one of the coagulation factors, also known as antihemophilic factor. Inherited deficiencies of this factor cause hemophilia A or classic hemophilia. Hemophilia B is a deficiency in Factor IX.

Febrile [L. *febrilis* fever] characterized or accompanied by fever.

Fibrin [L. *fibra* a fibre] the insoluble protein making up the long threads that bind a clot together.

Fibrinogen [Gr. *fibra* a fibre + *gen* to produce] One of the three major plasma proteins. In the clotting process fibrinogen is converted into insoluble strands of fibrin that bind the clot together.

Fibrinolysis [L. *fibra* a fibre + Gr. *lysis* dissolution] the dissolving of a blood clot by an enzyme that digests the fibrin that binds the clot.

Fractionation [L. *frangere, fractum* to break] the separation of a substance into its components.

Gynecology [Gr. *gyne* woman + *logos* study] the medical specialty dealing with diseases of the female genital tract and reproductive system; gynecologic surgery.

Hematocrit (Hct) [Gr. *haima* blood + *krino* to separate] a measurement of the percentage of red blood cells to the total blood volume.

Hematology [Gr. *haima* blood + *logos* study] the medical specialty that deals with the study of blood; its formation, diseases and related treatments.

Hematopoiesis, also **Hemopoiesis** [Gr. *haima* blood + *poiesis* making] the formation of blood.

Hemodilution [Gr. *haima* blood + *dilution* L. *diluere* to wash away] a decrease in the concentration of red blood cells by means of an increase in the fluid content of blood. Deliberate controlled hemodilution using intravenous fluids is a therapeutic strategy employed in surgery to reduce blood loss and allogeneic blood transfusion.

Hemoglobin (Hb) [Gr. *haima* blood + L. *globus* globule] the oxygen-carrying molecule in red blood cells.

Hemolysis [Gr. *haima* blood + *lysis* dissolution, destruction] The breakdown or destruction of red blood cells.

Hemolytic reaction a reaction in which red blood cells are destroyed.

Hemorrhage [Gr. *haima* blood + *rhegnymi* to burst forth] to bleed; blood escaping from the blood vessels.

Hemostasis [Gr. *haima* blood + *stasis* halt, a standing] the stopping of bleeding.

HIV human immunodificiency virus.

Homeostasis [Gr. *homoios* like or same + *stasis* standing] the maintenance of the body's internal environment in a balanced relatively constant state.

Homologous [Gr. *homologos* agreeing, corresponding] similarity in structure, position and origin. See allogeneic.

Hormones [Gr. *hormaein* to set in motion, spur on] substances produced by the body that control and regulate the function of organs. They bind to cells and speed up, slow down, or in some other way alter the cell's function, and so are like messengers that coordinate the activities of the body's various parts.

HTLV human T-cell lymphoma/leukemia virus.

Hyperoxic [Gr. *hyper* above, over + *oxygen*] relating to an increased amount of oxygen.

Hypotension [Gr. *hypo* under + *tension*] lower than normal blood pressure.

Hypotensive anesthesia or **controlled hypotension** is a lowering of the patient's blood pressure during surgery with medications or by anesthetic techniques in order to reduce bleeding.

Hypothermia [Gr. *hypo* under + *therme* heat + *ia* state] low body temperature. Sometimes deliberately induced as a means of slowing metabolism and reducing oxygen consumption in an anemic patient or used in combination with other techniques to perform major surgery. Needs to be used cautiously as hypothermia interferes with coagulation.

Idiopathic [Gr *idios* one's own, separate + *pathos* disease] used to describe a disease of unknown cause.

Immunodeficiency a deficient immune response.

Immunoglobulins [L. *immunis* free, exempt + *globulus* globule] One of the main plasma protein groups. Immunoglobulins are antibodies produced by plasma cells and B lymphocytes and form part of the body's immune system. There are many classes and subclasses of immunoglobulins.

Immunomodulation alteration of the immune response.

Immunosuppression inducing suppression of the immune response.

Infection [L. *inficere* to dip into] disease caused by the invasion and multiplication of microorganisms in body tissue.

Interleukins hormone-like substances that regulate immune responses and blood cell function, development and proliferation.

Latent [L. *latens* to lie hidden] dormant.

Leukocytes [Gr. *leukos* white + *kytos* cell] white blood cells of which there are five main types: neutrophils, monocytes, eosinophils, basophils and lymphocytes. Lymphocytes are further categorized as B lymphocytes, that develop into plasma cells and produce antibodies, and T lymphocytes.

Metabolism [Gr. *metaballein* to turn about, change, alter] All the chemical reactions of the body involved in the vital processes of life. Includes anabolism (Gr. *anabole* a throwing up) the combining of simple substances into more complex molecules for use by the body, and catabolism (Gr. *katabole* a throwing down) the breaking down of complex organic compounds into simple ones. Both processes involve an exchange of energy.

Meticulous hemostasis meticulous attention to preventing and stopping bleeding in the operating field. It requires a skilful and careful approach.

Microaggregates the collection or clumping of microscopic particles, such as platelets, white blood cells, fibrin and breakdown products in stored blood.

Morbidity [L. *morbidus* sick] a diseased or unhealthy condition or state.

Mortality [L. *mortalis* death] death or death-rate.

Multimodality [L. *multis* many + *modus* measure, manner, method] the application of many therapeutic methods, techniques, agents and devices.

Neonatology [Gr. *neos* new + L. *natus* born + Gr. *logos* study] the medical specialty (subspecialty of pediatrics) dealing with disorders of the newborn infant.

Neurology [Gr. *neuron* nerve + *logos* study] the medical specialty dealing with disorders of the nervous systems (including the brain and spinal cord); neurosurgery.

Obstetrics [L. *obstetrix* midwife, from *ob-sto* to stand before] the medical specialty that deals with women during pregnancy, birth and the period immediately following birth.

Orthopedics also **orthopaedics** [Gr. *ortho* correct, straight + *pais* child. The term originally applied to the curing or correcting of deformities in children and then extended to persons in general] the medical specialty that deals with the musculoskeletal (muscles and skeleton) system and associated structures; orthopedic surgery.

Parasites [Gr. *parasitos* one who eats at the table of another, from *para* beside + *sitos* food] a living organism that lives on or inside another organism.

Pathogens [Gr. *pathos* disease + *gen* to produce] any disease-producing organism.

Pediatrics [Gr. *pais* child + *iatreia* medical treatment] the medical specialty that deals with the treatment of children from birth through to adolescence; pediatric surgery.

Perfluorochemicals or **Perfluorocarbons** synthetic intravenous solutions that have the ability to carry oxygen. Not yet approved for general use.

Perioperative [Gr. *peri* around + *operation*] the period before, during and after surgery.

Plasma [Gr. *plasma* anything formed or molded] The fluid part of blood in which all the other components are suspended.

Platelets minute cell-like round or oval discs (deriving their name from their plate-like shape) in the blood that initiate and play a critical role in the blood clotting process.

Prions infectious particles thought to be the cause of degenerative nerve diseases such as Creutzfeldt-Jakob disease.

Purpura [L. *purpura* purple] purplish spots on the skin as a result of bleeding from the capillaries into the skin.

Recombinant [from recombine] artificially constructed by genetic engineering.

Sequestration [L. *sequestrare* to lay aside or, to put in safe keeping] In medicine, the process of separating a small portion from the whole.

Stem cells or more specifically, **hemopoietic stem cells** the common "mother" or progenitor cells in the bone marrow from which all blood cells originate.

Storage lesion [*storage* + L. *laesio/laedere* to hurt] A term used to describe the physical and chemical changes blood undergoes during storage.

Thoracic [Gr. *thorax* breastplate, the chest] pertaining to the thorax or chest; the upper part of the trunk of the body, between the abdomen (diaphragm) and the neck, containing the main organs of the circulatory and respiratory systems; thoracic surgeon.

Thrombocytes [Gr. *thrombos* clot + *kylos* cell] blood platelets.

Thrombocytopenia [*thrombocyte* + Gr. *penia* poverty] deficiency of platelets in blood.

Thrombopoietin a hormone that stimulates the formation of platelets.

Toxin [Gr. *toxikon* poison] A poisonous substance.

Transfusion [L. *trans* across + *fundere/fusum* to pour] Literally, transferring liquid from one vessel to another and used generally for the introducing of fluids into a vein.

Ventilator a mechanical device used to assist breathing by forcing air into the lungs.

Viruses [L. *virus* poison] Viruses are tiny infectious organisms, much smaller than bacteria. They are not able to replicate on their own, but require other living host cells to reproduce. Once inside a cell the virus releases its DNA or RNA and takes over control of some aspects of the cell's function. Like bacteria, viruses come in different shapes but are classified according to their preferred host, their origin, method of transmission, their effects or geographical location of their discovery.

Volume expanders a range of synthetic fluids used to replace lost blood volume.

White blood cells see Leukocytes.

Please note: In the UK, Australia and other parts of the English speaking world, words such as hematology, gynecology, orthopedics, etc., are spelt haematology, gynaecology and orthopaedics.

Sources: Stedman's Medical Dictionary 26th Edition. Dorland's Illustrated Medical Dictionary 27th Edition. Principles of Anatomy and Physiology 8th Edition. Mosby's Medical, Nursing, & Allied Health Dictionary. 5th Edition. The Merck Manual of Medical Information: Home Edition. Essential Haematology 3rd Edition. Harrison's Principles of Internal Medicine 12th Edition. The Compact Edition of The Oxford English Dictionary.

APPENDIX 5

Bibliography / References

Chapter 1

Seu P, Neelankanta G, Csete M, et al. Liver transplantation for fulminant hepatic failure in a Jehovah's Witness. *Clin Transplantation* 1996;10:404-407.

Ramos HC, Todo S, Kang Y, et al. Liver Transplantation Without the Use of Blood Products. *Arch Surg* 1994;129:528-33.

Walker RH. Is it homologous or is it allogeneic? *Transfusion* 1992;32(5):397-8.

Cooley DA, Crawford ES, Howell JF, Beall AC jr. Open Heart Surgery in Jehovah's Witnesses. *Am J Cardiology* 1964;13:779-781.

Ott DA, Cooley DA. Cardiovascular Surgery in Jehovah's Witnesses: Report of 542 Operations Without Blood Transfusion. *JAMA* 1977;238:1256-1258.

Henling CE, Carmichael MJ, Keats AS, Cooley DA. Cardiac operation for congenital heart disease in children of Jehovah's Witnesses. *J Thorac Cardiovasc Surg* 1985;89:914-920.

Carmichael MJ, Cooley DA, Kuykendall RC, Walker WE. Cardiac Surgery in Children of Jehovah's Witnesses. *Texas Heart Institute Journal* 1985;12(1):57-63.

Cooley DA. Conservation of Blood During Cardiovascular Surgery. *Am J Surg* 1995;170(suppl 6A):53S-59S.

Gollub S, Bailey CP. Management of Major Surgical Blood Loss Without Transfusion. *JAMA* 1966;198(11):1171-1174.

Bailey CP, Hirose T, Gollub S, et al. Open Heart Surgery Without Blood Transfusion. *Vascular Diseases* 1968;5(4):179-187.

Kay JH. Need for Blood in Open-Heart Surgery. *JAMA* 1973;226(10):1230.

Kawaguchi A, Bergsland J, Subramanian S. Total bloodless open heart surgery in the pediatric age group. *Circulation* 1984;70(suppl 1):1.30-1.37.

Nelson CL, Martin K, Lawson N, et al. Total Hip Replacement Without Transfusion. *Contemporary Orthopaedics* 1980;2(9):655-658.

Alexiu O, Mircea N, Balaban M, Furtunescu B. Gastro-intestinal haemorrhage from peptic ulcer: An evaluation of bloodless transfusion and early surgery. *Anaesthesia* 1975;30:609-615.

Kambouris AA. Major Abdominal Operations on Jehovah's Witnesses. *Am Surg* 1987;6:350-356.

Phillips WA, Hensinger RN. Control of Blood Loss During Scoliosis Surgery. *Clinical Orthopaedics and Related Research* 1988;229:88-93.

Polk HC, Garrison JR. Blood Management Practice Guidelines: Conference Highlights. *Am J Surg* 1995;170(suppl 6A):1S-2S.

Garcia F, Juri H, Lapin R. Anemia and Anesthesia. *J Bloodless Med & Surgery* 1986;4(1):15-18.

Garcia F, Lapin R, Corssen G. General Anesthesia for the Anemic Patient Without Blood Therapy. *J Bloodless Med & Surgery* 1983:20-23.

Lapin R. Major Surgery in Jehovah's Witnesses. *Contemporary Orthopaedics* 1980;2(9):647-654.

Belghiti J. Ethical Aspects of Bloodless Surgery: The Surgeon's Viewpoint. In: Belghiti J, Castot M, Conseiller C, et al., editors. *Bloodless Surgery: Surgical and Anaesthetic Aspects; Legal and Ethical Issues.* Paris: Arnette Blackwell; 1997:141-142.

Roberts HR. The Treatment of Hemophilia – Past Tragedy and Future Promise. *N Eng J Med* 1989;321(17):1188-1190.

Schlagintweit S, Snelling CFT, Germann E, et al. Major Burns Managed Without Blood or Blood Products. *J Burn Care Rehabil* 1990;11:214-220.

Moghtader JC, Edlich RF, Mintz PD, Zachmann GC, Himel HN. The use of recombinant human erythropoietin and cultured epithelial autografts in a Jehovah's Witness with a major thermal injury. *Burns* 1994:20(2):176-177.

McGill V, Kowal-Vern A, Gamelli RL. A conservative thermal injury treatment protocol for the appropriate Jehovah's Witness candidate. *J Burn Care Rehab* 1997;18(2):133-138.

Donner B, Tryba M, Kurz-Muller K, et al. Anesthesia and intensive care management of severely burned children of Jehovah's Witnesses. *Anaesthesist* 1996;45(2):171-175.

Dor V, Montiglio F, Quaegebeur J. Bloodless Adult and Paediatric Cardiac Surgery with Cardiopulmonary Bypass. In: Belghiti J, Castot M, Conseiller C, et al., editors. *Bloodless Surgery: Surgical and Anaesthetic Aspects; Legal and Ethical Issues.* Paris; Arnette Blackwell, 1997:63-72.

Estioko MR, Litwak RS, Rand JH. Reoperation, emergency and urgent open cardiac surgery in Jehovah's Witnesses. *Chest* 1992;102(1):50-53.

Helm RE, Rosengart TK, Gomez M, Klemperer JD, DeBois WJ, Velasco F, Gold JP. Comprehensive multimodality blood conservation: 100 consecutive CABG operations without transfusion. *Ann Thorac Surg* 1998;65(1):125-136.

Kemp G, Rose P, Lurain J, Berman M, Manetta A, Roullet B, et al. Amifostine pretreatment for protection against cyclophosphamide-induced and cisplatin-induced toxicities: results of a randomized control trial in patients with advanced ovarian cancer. *J Clin Oncol* 1996;14(7):2101-2112.

Schaller RT jr, Schaller J, Morgan A, Furman EB. Hemodilution Anesthesia: A Valuable Aid to Major Cancer Surgery in Children. *Am J Surg* 1983;146:79-84.

Adzick NS, deLorimier AA, Harrison MR, et al. Major Childhood Tumor Resection Using Normovolemic Hemodilution Anesthesia and Hetastarch. *Journal of Pediatric Surgery* 1985;20(4):372-375.

Schaller RT jr, Schaller J, Furman EB. The Advantages of Hemodilution Anesthesia for Major Liver Resection in Children. *Journal of Pediatric Surgery* 1984;19(6):705-710.

MacMillan ML, Freedman MH. Recombinant human erythropoietin in children with cancer. *Pediatr Hematol Oncol* 1998;20(3):187-189.

Atabek U, Spence RK, Pello M, Alexander J, Camishion R. Pancreaticoduodenectomy without homologous blood transfusion in an anemic Jehovah's Witness. *Arch Surg* 1992;127(3):349-351.

So SK, Monge H, Esquivel CO. Major hepatic resection without blood transfusion: experience with total vascular exclusion. *J Gastroenterol Hepatol* 1999; 14 (Suppl):S28-S31.

Fan ST, Lo CM, Liu CL, et al. Hepatectomy for hepatocellular carcinoma: toward zero hospital deaths. *Ann Surg* 1999;229(3):322-330.

Thomas MJG. Infected and malignant fields are an absolute contraindication to intraoperative cell salvage: fact or fiction? *Transfus Med* 1999;9(3):269-278.

McGehee RP, Dodson MK, Moore JL, Morrison FS, Bass JD, Burrow P, Morrison JC. Effect of blood transfusion in patients with gynecologic malignancy. *Int J Gynecol Obst* 1994;46(1):45-52.

Powell JL, Mogelnicki SR, Franklin EW, et al. A deliberate hypotensive technique for decreasing blood loss during radical hysterectomy and pelvic lymphadenectomy. *Am J Obstet Gynecol* 1983;147(2):196-202.

Bonakdar MI, Eckhous AW, Bacher BJ, et al. Major Gynecologic and Obstetric Surgery in Jehovah's Witnesses. *Obstet Gynecol* 1982;60(5):587-590.

Estrin JT, Ford PA, Henry DH, Stradden AP, Mason BA. Erythropoietin permits high-dose chemotherapy with peripheral blood stem-cell transplant for a Jehovah's Witness. *Am J Hematol* 1997;55(1):51-52.

Kerridge I, Lowe M, Seldon M, Enno A, Deveridge S. Clinical and ethical issues in the treatment of a Jehovah's Witness with acute myeloblastic leukemia. *Arch Intern Med* 1997;157(15):1753-1757.

Fernandes CJ, Hagan R, Frieberg A, Grauaug A, Kohan R. Erythropoietin in very preterm infants. *J Paediatr Child Health* 1994;30:356-359.

Ohls RK, Harcum J, Schibler KR, Christensen RD. The effect of erythropoietin on the transfusion requirements of preterm infants weighing 750 grams or less: a randomized, double-blind, placebo-controlled study. *J Pediatr* 1997;131(5):661-665.

Garland JS, Alex CP, Pauly TH, Whitehead VL, Brand J, Winston JF, et al. A three-day course of dexamethasone therapy to prevent chronic lung disease in ventilated neonates: a randomized trial. *Pediatrics* 1999;104(1 Pt 1):91-99.

Donzelli GP, Moroni M, Pratesi S, Rapisardi G, Agati G, Fusi F. Fibreoptic phototherapy in the management of jaundice in low birthweight neonates. *Acta Paediatr* 1996;85(3):366-370.

Martinez JC, Garcia HO, Otheguy LE, Drummond GS, Kappas A. Control of severe hyperbilirubinemia in full-term newborns with the inhibitor of bilirubin production Sn-mesoporphyrin. *Pediatrics* 1999;103(1):1-5.

Posnikoff J. Cure of Intracranial Aneurysm Without Use of Blood Transfusion. *California Medicine* 1967;106(2):124-127.

Kantrowitz AB, Spallone A, Taylor W, et al. Erythropoietin-augmented isovolemic hemodilution in skull-base surgery. *J Neurosurg* 1994;80:740-744.

Kondziolka D, Lunsford LD, McLaughlin MR, Flickinger JC. Long-term outcomes after radiosurgery for acoustic neuromas. *N Engl J Med* 1998;339(20):1426-1433.

Drife J. Management of primary post partum haemorrhage. *Br J Obstet Gynaecol* 1997;104(3):275-277.

Thomas JM. The treatment of obstetric haemorrhage in women who refuse blood transfusion. *Br J Obstet Gynaecol* 1998;105(1):127-128.

Rebarber A, Lonser R, Jackson S, Copel JA, Sipes S. The safety of intraoperative autologous blood collection and autotransfusion during cesarean section. *Am J Obstet Gynecol*

1998;179(3 Pt 1):715-720.

Breymann C, Zimmerman R, Huch R, Huch A. Use of recombinant human erythropoietin in combination with parenteral iron in the treatment of postpartum anemia. *Eur J Clin Invest* 1996;26(2):123-130.

Hudon L, Belfort MA, Broome DR. Diagnosis and management of placenta percreta: a review. *Obstet Gynecol Surg* 1998;53(8):509-517.

Mitty HA, Sterling KM, Alvarez M, et al. Obstetric hemorrhage: prophylactic and emergency arterial catheterization and embolotherapy. *Radiology* 1993;188(1):183-7.

Nelson CL, Fontenot HJ. Ten strategies to reduce blood loss in orthopedic surgery. *Am J Surg* 1995;170(6a Suppl):64S-68S.

deAndrade JR. Prudent strategies for red cell conservation in orthopedic surgery. *Am J Med* 1996;101(suppl 2A):16S-21S.

Meyers MO, Heinrich S, Kline R, Levine EA. Extended hemipelvectomy in a Jehovah's Witness with erythropoietin support. *Am Surg* 1998;64(11):1074-1076.

Hur SR, Huizenga BA, Major M. Acute normovolemic hemodilution combined with hypotensive anesthesia and other techniques to avoid homologous transfusion in spinal fusion surgery. *Spine* 1992;17(8):867-887.

Dupuis JF, Nguyen DT. Anesthetic Management of the Patient Who Refuses Blood Transfusion. *The Cancer Bulletin* 1995;47(1):67-73.

Son JAM, Hovaguimian H, Rao IM, He GW, Meiling GA, King DH, Starr A. Strategies for repair of congenital heart defects in infants without the use of blood. *Ann Thorac Surg* 1995;59:384-388.

Kerman RH, Van Buren CT, Lewis RM, Kahan BD. Successful Transplantation of 100 Untransfused Cyclosporine-Treated Primary Recipients of Cadaveric Renal Allografts. *Transplantation* 1988;45(1):37-40

Kaufman DB, Sutherland DE, Fryd DS, Ascher NL, Simmons RL, Najarian JS. A single-center experience of renal transplantation in thirteen Jehovah's Witnesses. *Transplantation* 1988;45(6):1045-1049.

Potter PS. Utilization of Autologous Transfusion Technologies for Allogeneic-blood-free Cardiac Transplantation in Pediatric Patients. *TATM* 1999;1(1):26-28.

Burnett CM, Duncan JM, Vega JD, Lonquist JL, Sweeney MS, Frazier OH. Heart transplantation in Jehovah's Witnesses. An initial experience and follow-up. *Arch Surg* 1990;125(11):1430-1433.

Snook NJ, O'Beirne HA, Enright S, et al. Use of recombinant human erythropoietin to facilitate liver transplantation in a Jehovah's Witness. *Br J Anaesth* 1996;76(5):740-743.

Conte JV, Orens JB. Lung transplantation in a Jehovah's Witness. *J Heart Lung Transplantation* 1999;18(8):796-800.

Losty PD, Okoye BO, Walter DP, Turnock RR, Lloyd DA. Management of blunt liver trauma in children. *Br J Surg* 1997;84(7):1006-1008.

Zantut LFC, Machado MAC, Volpe P, Poggetti RS, Birolini D. Autotransfusion with laparoscopically salvaged blood in trauma: report on 21 cases. *Surg Laparosc Endosc* 1996;6(1):46-48.

Moore EE, Burch JM, Franciose RJ, Offner PJ, Biffl WL. Staged physiologic restoration and damage control surgery. *World J Surg* 1998;22(12):1184-1191.

Roen PR, Velcek F. Extensive Urologic Surgery Without Blood Transfusion. *New York State Journal of Medicine* 1972:2524-2527.

Hill I. The Harmonic Scalpel in Radical Prostatectomy. *Bloodless Surgery Update* 1998;3(1):1.

Westaby S, Parry AJ, Lamont P, Grebenik C. Massive Descending Thoracic Aneurysm in a Jehovah's Witness: Treatment by Thromboexclusion. *Ann Thorac Surg* 1993;55:1233-1235.

Chapter 2

Hoffbrand AV, Pettit JE, editors. *Essential Haematology,* 3rd ed. Blackwell Science; 1993.

Tortora GJ, Anagnostakos NP, editors. *Principles of Anatomy and Physiology,* 8th ed. Addison-Wesley; 1996.

Wilson JD, Braunwald E, Isselbacher KJ, et al., editors. *Harrison's Principles of Internal Medicine,* 14th ed. McGraw Hill; 1997.

Spraycar M, Randolph E, Pugh MB, et al., editors. *Stedman's Medical Dictionary*, 26th ed. Williams & Wilkins; 1995.

Myhre BA. The first recorded blood transfusions: 1656 to 1668. *Transfusion* 1990;30(4):358-362.

Spence RK, Cernaianu AC, Carson J, et al. Transfusion and Surgery. *Curr Probl Surg* 1993;30(12):1103-1180.

Bibb LM, Nimmagadda U, Mastrianno L. Principles of Blood Transfusion. In: Salem MR, editor. *Blood Conservation in the Surgical Patient.* Baltimore: Williams & Wilkins; 1996:1-44.

Zauder HL, Stehling L. History and Development of Transfusion Medicine. In: Stehling L, Spence R, Contreras M, et al. Editors. *Transfusion Medicine and Alternatives to Blood Transfusion.* Paris: R&J Éditions Médicales; 2000:11-19.

Starr D. *Blood: An Epic History of Medicine and Commerce.* New York: Alfred A. Knopf; 1998.

Farmer DF. Transfusion of Cadaver Blood: A Contribution to the History of Blood Transfusion. *Bulletin of the American Association of Blood Banks.* 1960:229-234.

Vyas GN, Munver UL, Salgaonkar DS, Purandare NM. Human Cadaver Blood for Transfusion. *Transfusion* 1968;(8):250-253.

Kevorkian J, Bylsma GW. Transfusion of Postmortem Human Blood. *Am J Clin Pathol* 1961;35:413-419

Kevorkian J, Marra JJ. Transfusion of Human Corpse Blood Without Additives. *Transfusion* 1964;(4):112-117

Chapter 3 (Including Appendix I)

Beeson PB. Jaundice occurring one to four months after transfusion of blood or plasma. *JAMA* 1943;121:1332.

Jackson JO. Scandal in Red. *Time* November 15, 1993:24-29.

Pincock S. Investigating the Bringer of Life and Death. Today's *Life Science* September 1995:78-80.

Commission of Inquiry on the Blood System in Canada. Interim report. Ottawa: Canadian Government Publishing-PWGSC; 1995.

Commission of Inquiry on the Blood System in Canada. Final report. Ottawa: Canadian Government Publishing-PWGSC; 1997. Available from: URL: http://www.hc-sc.ca/english/krever/

Avoy DR. Private Enterprise, Nontraditional Blood Banking. In: Garner RJ, Silvergleid AJ, editors. *Autologous and Directed Blood Programs* Arlington, VA: American Association of Blood Banks; 1987:65-66.

Desposito F, McSherry GD, Oleske JM. Blood Product Acquired HIV Infection in Children *Pediatric Annals* 1988;17(5):341-345.

Salzberg, et al. Transmission of HIV by Blood Transfusion. *N Engl J Med* 1988;319:513.

Haseltine. Silent HIV Infections. *N Engl J Med* 1989;320:1487.

Imagawa DT, Lee MH, Wolinsky SM, et al. Human Immunodeficiency Virus Type 1 Infection in Homosexual Men Who Remain Seronegative for Prolonged Periods. *N Engl J Med* 1989;320(22):1458-1462.

Ward JW, Holmberg SD, Allen JR, et al. Transmission of Human Immunodificiency Virus (HIV) by Blood Transfusions Screened as Negative for HIV Antibody. *N Engl J Med* 1988;318(8):473-478.

Cohen ND, Munoz A, Reitz BA, et al. Transmission of Retroviruses by Transfusion of Screened Blood in Patients Undergoing Cardiac Surgery. *N Engl J Med* 1989;320:1172-1176.

Sandler SG. HTLV-I and –II: New Risks for Recipients of Blood Transfusions? *JAMA* 1986;256(16):2245-2246

Aboulafia DM. Clinical Implications of Human T-Cell Leukemia Virus type I/II – Associated Diseases. *The AIDS Reader* 1995;5(4):118-135.

Loussert-Ajaka I, Ly TD, Chaix ML, et al. HIV-1/HIV-2 seronegativity in HIV-1 subtype O infected patients. *Lancet* 1994;343:1393-1394.

Schuttler CG, Caspari G, Jursch CA, et al. Hepatitis C virus transmission by a blood donation negative in nucleic acid amplification tests for viral RNA. *Lancet* 2000;355(9197):41-42.

Dodd RY. The risk of transfusion-transmitted infection. *N Engl J Med* 1992;327:419-420.

Ereth MH. Perioperative interventions to decrease transfusions of allogeneic blood products. *Mayo Clinic Proceedings* 1994;69:575-586.

Friedrich MJ. Third Millennium Challenge: Hepatitis C. *JAMA* 1999;282(3):221-222.

Bowden DS, et al. New hepatitis viruses are there enough letters in the alphabet? *Med J Aust* 1995;164:87-89.

Shafran SD, Conly JM. Adult Infectious Disease Notes. ABCDEFG . . . *Can J Infect Dis* 1996;7(3):181-182.

Gordon SC, Elloway RS, Long JC, Dmuchowski CF. The pathology of hepatitis C as a function of mode of transmission: blood transfusion vs. intravenous drug use. *Hepatology* 1993;18(6):1338-1343.

Hepatitis C: A Challenge to Public Health. *Congressional Research Service Report to Congress.* The Library of Congress; March 4, 1998.

Orii K, Tanaka E. Non A-G chronic hepatitis in Japan. *Nippon Rinsho* 1999;57(6):1269-1273.

Chamberland M, Khabbaz RF. Emerging Issues in Blood Safety. *Infectious Disease Clinics of North America* 1998;12(1):217-229.

Chamberland ME, Epstein J, Dodd RY, et al. Blood safety. *Emerg Infect Dis* 1998;4(3):410-411.

Allain JP. Emerging viruses in blood transfusion. *Vox Sang* 1998;74(suppl 2):125-129.

Inaba S. Severe complications, adverse effects due to blood transfusion and its measures – transfusion transmitted viral infections. *Nippon Rinsho* 1997;55(9):2320-2326.

Thomas DP. Viral contamination of blood products. *Lancet* 1994;343(8913):1583-1584.

Charlton M, Adjei P, Poterucha J, et al. TT-Virus Infection in North American Blood Donors, Patients With Fulminant Hepatic Failure, and Cryptogenic Cirrhosis. *Hepatology* 1998;28:839-842.

Kobayashi M, Chayama K, Arase Y, et al. Prevalence of TT virus before and after blood transfusion in patients with chronic liver disease treated surgically for hepatocellular carcinoma. *J Gastroenterol Hepatol* 1999;14(4):358-363.

Fernandez Lopez MJ, Van Everbroeck B, Pals P, et al. Creutzfeldt-Jakob disease and blood transfusion. *Eur J Haematol* 1999;62(1):1-18.

Turner ML, Ironside JW. New-variant Creutzfeldt-Jakob disease: the risk of transmission by blood transfusion. *Acta Neurol Belg* 1998;98(3):247-251.

Collinge J. Variant Creutzfeldt-Jakob disease. *Lancet* 1999;354(9175):317-323.

Tartter P. Is the blood transfusion effect real? *J Intensive Care Med* 1992;7:167-169.

Blumberg N. Allogeneic Transfusion and Infection: Economic and Clinical Implications. *Seminars in Hematology* 1997;34(3 suppl 2):34-40.

Blumberg N, Heal JM. Immunomodulation by Blood Transfusion: An Evolving Scientific and Clinical Challenge. *Am J Med* 1996;101:299-308.

Blumberg N, Heal JM. Blood Transfusion Immunomodulation – The Silent Epidemic. *Arch Pathol Lab Med* 1998;122:117-119.

Kirkley SA, Blumberg N. Increased Postoperative Infections after Transfusion of Allogeneic Blood. In: Tawes RL Jr., ed. *Autotransfusion: Therapeutic Principles and Trends.* Detroit: Gregory Appleton;1997:368-373.

Carson JL, Altman DG, Duff A, et al. Risk of bacterial infection associated with allogeneic blood transfusion among patients undergoing hip fracture repair. *Transfusion* 1999;39:694-700.

Murphy P, Heal JM, Blumberg N. Infection or suspected infection after hip replacement surgery with autologous or homologous blood transfusions. *Transfusion* 1991;31:212-217.

Michalopoulos A, Tzelepis G, Dafni U, Geroulanos S. Determinants of Hospital Mortality After Coronary Artery Bypass Grafting. *Chest* 1999;115:1598-1603.

Mudido PM, Georges D, Dorazio D, et al. Human immunodeficiency virus type 1 activation after blood transfusion. *Transfusion* 1996;36(10):860-865.

Blajchman MA. Transfusion-associated immunomodulation and universal white cell reduction: are we putting the cart before the horse? *Transfusion* 1999;39:665-669.

Tartter PI. The Association of Perioperative Blood Transfusion With Colorectal Cancer Recurrence *Ann Surg* 1992;216(6):633-638.

Vamvakas EC. Perioperative blood transfusion and cancer recurrence. *Transfusion* 1995;35:760-768.

Blumberg N, Agarwal MM, Chuang C. Relationship between recurrence of cancer of the colon and blood transfusion. *Br Med J* 1985;290:1037-1039.

Eisenkop SM, Spirtos NM, Montag TW, et al. The Clinical Significance of Blood Transfusion at the Time of Radical Hysterectomy. *Obstet Gynecol* 1990;76(1):110-113.

Tartter PI, Burrows L, Papatestas AE, et al. Perioperative blood transfusion has prognostic significance for breast cancer. *Surgery* 1985;97(2):225-230.

Eroglu A, Canpinar H, Kansu E. Influence of perioperative whole blood transfusions on lymphocyte subpopulations in patients with stage II breast cancer. *Med Oncol* 1999;16(1):53-57.

Rosenberg SA, Seipp CA, White DE, Wesley R. Perioperative blood transfusions are associated with increased rates of recurrence and decreased survival in patients with high-grade soft-tissue sarcomas of the extremities. *J Clin Oncol* 1985;3:698-709.

Chesi R, Cazzola A, Bacci G, et al. Effect of perioperative transfusions on survival in osteosarcoma treated by multimodal therapy. *Cancer* 1989;64(8):1727-1737.

Moores DWO, Piantadosi S, McKneally MF. Effect of Perioperative Blood Transfusion on Outcome in Patients With Surgically Resected Lung Cancer. *Ann Thorac Surg* 1989;47:346-351.

Little AG, Wu HS, Ferguson MK, et al. Perioperative blood transfusion adversely affects prognosis of patients with stage I non-small-cell lung cancer. *Am J Surg* 1990;160(6):630-632.

Heal JM, Chuang C, Blumberg N. Perioperative blood transfusion and prostate cancer recurrence and survival. *Am J Surg* 1988;156:374.

Jackson RM, Rice DH, Blood transfusion and recurrence in head and neck cancer. *Ann Otol Laryngol* 1989;90:171-173.

Moir MS, Samy RN, Hanasono MM, Terris DJ. Autologous and heterologous blood transfusion in head and neck cancer surgery. *Arch Otolaryngol Head Neck Surg* 1999;125(8):864-868.

Asahara T, Katayama K, Itamoto T, et al. Perioperative blood transfusion as a prognostic indicator in patients with hepatocellular carcinoma. *World J Surg* 1999;23(7):676-680.

Tachibana M, Tabara H, Kotoh T, et al. Prognostic significance of perioperative blood transfusions in resectable thoracic esophageal cancer. *Am J Gastroenterol* 1999;94(3):757-765.

Tartter PI. Clinical Studies of Blood Transfusion and Cancer Recurrence. In: Tartter PI. *Medical Intelligence Unit. Immunologic Aspects of Blood Transfusion.* Austin / Georgetown, TX: RG Landes Company 1992; pp. 54-81.

Spratt JS. Blood transfusions and surgery for cancer. *Am J Surg* 1986; 152(3):337.

Fransen E, Maessen J, Dentener M, et al. Impact of Blood Transfusions on Inflammatory Mediator Release in Patients Undergoing Cardiac Surgery. *Chest* 1999;116:1233-1239.

Tartter PI, Mohandas K, Azar P, et al. Randomized Trial Comparing Packed Red Cell Blood Transfusion with and without Leukocyte Depletion for Gastrointestinal Surgery. *Am J Surg* 1998;176:462-466.

Lawrence-Brown MMD, Sieunarine K, Hellings M. The Non-Red Cell Elements in Blood for Transfusion. In: Tawes RL Jr., ed. *Autotransfusion: Therapeutic Principles and Trends.* Detroit: Gregory Appleton;1997:329-338.

Sieunarine K, Lawrence-Brown MMD, Brennan D, et al. The quality of blood used for transfusion. *J Cardiovasc Surg* 1992;33(1):98-105.

Chin-Yee I, Arya N, d'Almeida MS. The red cell storage lesion and its implication for transfusion. *Transfus Sci* 1997; 18(3); 447-58.

Sugerman JH, Davidson DT, Vibul S, et al. The basis of defective oxygen delivery from stored blood. *Surgical Gynecology and Obstetrics* 1970;137:733-741.

McConn R, Derrick JB. The respiratory function of blood: transfusion and blood storage. *Anesthesiology* 1972;36:119-127.

Jesch F, Webber LM, Dalton JW. Oxygen dissociation after transfusion of blood stored in ACD or CPD solution. *J Thorac Cardiovasc Surg* 1975;70:35-39.

Haradin AR, Weed RI, Reed CF. Changes in physical properties of stored erythrocytes. Relationship to survival *in vivo. Transfusion* 1969;9:238-245.

LaCelle PL. Alterations of deformability of the erythrocyte membrane in stored blood. *Transfusion* 1969;9:238-245.

Allen JB, Allen FB. The Minimum Acceptable Level of Hemoglobin. *International Anesthesiology Clinics* 1982;20(4):1-22.

Vamvakas EC, Carven JH. Transfusion and postoperative pneumonia in coronary artery bypass surgery: effect of the length of storage on transfused red cells. *Transfusion* 1999;39:701-710.

Linden JV. Errors in transfusion medicine. Scope of the problem. *Arch Pathol Lab Med* 1999;123(7):563-565.

Williams L. Homologous Blood Transfusion: The Risk and Alternatives. *British Journal of Haematology* 1994;88(3):451-458.

Isbister J. Risk Management in Transfusion Medicine. *Transfusion Medicine Reviews* 1996;10(3):183-202.

Hardy JF. Blood products: when to use them and how to avoid them. *Canadian Journal of Anaesthesia* 1994;41(suppl Pt 2):R52-R61.

Pink JM, Isbister JP. What's new in clinical transfusion practice. *Med J Aust* 1996;165:30-34.

Bibb LM, Nimmagadda U, Mastrianno. Principles of Blood Transfusion. In: Salem MR, editor. *Blood Conservation in the Surgical Patient.* Baltimore: Williams & Wilkins; 1996:1-44.

Wilson JD, Braunwald E, Isselbacher KJ, et al., editors. *Harrison's Principles of Internal Medicine,* 14th ed. McGraw Hill; 1997.

Rossi, Simon, Moss, editors. *Principles of Transfusion Medicine.* Williams & Wilkins; 1991.

Circular of Information. An Extension of Blood and Component Container Labels. Australian Red Cross Blood Service, 1998.

Contreras M, editor. *ABC of Transfusion,* 3rd ed. BMJ Books; 1998.

British Committee for Standards in Haematology, Blood Transfusion Task Force in collaboration with the Royal College of Nursing and the Royal College of Surgeons of

England. The administration of blood and blood components and the management of transfused patients. *Transfusion Medicine* 1999;9:227-238.

Huston P, editor. *Building a Blood System for the 21st Century. Proceedings and Recommendations.* Symposium on blood transfusion and the medical alternatives; 1997 Nov 3-4; Toronto, Canada. Ottawa: Health Canada (Canadian Federal Ministry of Health)/ Canadian Blood Agency/Canadian Hemophilia Society; 1997.

Klein HG. New Insights into the Management of Anemia in the Surgical Patient. *Am J Med* 1996;101(suppl 2A):12S-15S.

Klein HG. Allogeneic Transfusion Risks in the Surgical Patient. *Am J Surg* 1995;170(suppl 6A):21S-26S.

Peters H. Adverse effects of allogeneic blood transfusion. *Erythropoiesis: New Dimensions in the Treatment of Anaemia* 1997;8:3-11.

Walker RH. Special Report: Transfusion Risks. *Am J Clin Pathol* 1987;88:374-378.

Heiss MM. Risk of allogeneic transfusions. *Br J Anaesth* 1998;81(suppl 1):16-19.

Goodnough LT, Brecher ME, Kanter MH, AuBuchon JP. Transfusion Medicine – Blood Transfusion. *N Engl J Med* 1999;340(6):438-446.

Maitani S, Nishikawa T, Hirakawa A, Tobe T. Role of Blood Transfusion in Organ System Failure Following Major Abdominal Surgery. *Ann Surg* 1986;203(3):275-281.

Moore FA, Moore EE, Sauaia A. Blood transfusion: An independent risk factor for postinjury multiple organ failure. *Arch Surg* 1997;132(6):620-4.

Chapter 4

Arnoux R, Corman J, Peloquin A, et al. Adverse Effect of Blood Transfusions on Patient Survival After Resection of Rectal Cancer. *Can J Surg* 1988;31(2):121-126.

Zauder HL. How Did We Get a "Magic Number" for Preoperative Hematocrit/Hemoglobin Level? Perioperative Red Cell Transfusion NIH Consensus Development Conference June 27-29, 1988. *Program and Abstracts.*

Eiseman B. Perioperative Blood Transfusion. *Surgical Rounds* 1988:31-40

National Institutes of Health Consensus Conference. Perioperative red blood cell transfusion. *JAMA* 1988;260(18):2700-2703

Welch JG, Meehan KR, Goodnough LT. Prudent Strategies for Elective Red Blood Cell Transfusion. *Ann Intern Med* 1992;116(5):393-402.

American College of Physicians. Clinical Guideline: Practice Strategies for Elective Red Blood Cell Transfusion. *Ann Intern Med* 1992;116(5):403-406.

Practice Guidelines for Blood Component Therapy: A Report by the American Society of Anesthesiologists Task Force on Blood Component Therapy. *Anesthesiology* 1996;84(3):732-747.

Simon TL, Alverson DC, AuBuchon J, et al. Practice Parameter for the Use of Red Blood Cell Transfusions. Developed by the Red Blood Cell Administration Practice Guideline Development Task Force of the College of American Pathologists. *Arch Pathol Lab Med* 1998;122:130-138.

Spence RK. Introduction. Proceedings of a Symposium: New Insights Into The Management of Anemia in the Surgical Patient. *Am J Med* 1996;101(suppl 2A):1S-3S.

Spence RK for the Blood Management Practice Guidelines Conference. Surgical Red Blood Cell Transfusion Practice Policies. *Am J Surg* 1995;170(suppl 6A):3S-15S.

Goodnough LT, Despotis GJ. Establishing Practice Guidelines for Surgical Blood Management. *Am J Surg* 1995;170(suppl 6A):16S-20S.

Ely EW, Bernard GR. Transfusion in Critically Ill Patients. *N Engl J Med* 1999;340(6):467-468.

Rosengart TK, Helm RE, DeBois WJ, et al. Open Heart Operations Without Transfusion Using a Multimodality Blood Conservation Strategy in 50 Jehovah's Witness Patients: Implications for a "Bloodless" Surgical Technique. *J Am Coll Surg* 1997;184:618-692.

Helm RE, Rosengart TK, Gomez M, et al. Comprehensive Multimodality Blood Conservation: 100 Consecutive CABG Operations Without Transfusion. *Ann Thorac Surg* 1998;65:125-136.

Vamvakas EC, Carven JH. Allogeneic Blood Transfusion, Hospital Charges, and Length of Hospitalization. A Study of 487 Consecutive Patients Undergoing Colorectal Cancer Resection. *Arch Pathol Lab Med* 1998;122:145-151.

Sculco TP. Blood Management in Orthopedic Surgery. *Am J Surg* 1995;170(6A Suppl):60S-63S.

Weiskopf R. More on the Changing Indications for Transfusion of Blood and Blood Components during Anesthesia. *Anesthesiology* 1996;84(3):498-501.

Ramsay S, Birchard K, Watts J. Variant CJD fears prompt growing number of countries to ban British blood donations. *Lancet* 1999;354(9180):754.

Franklin IM. The impact of British blood services on BSE and v-CJD: implications for patients, donors and public health. *Scott Med J* 1999; 44(2):35-36.

Muñoz E. The Hidden Costs of Homologous Blood. *Toltzis Communications, Inc;* 1991.

Blumberg N, Kirkely SA, Heal JM. A Cost Analysis of Autologous and Allogeneic Transfusions in Hip-Replacement Surgery. *Am J Surg* 1996;171:324-330.

Murphy PJ, et al. Homologous blood transfusions as a risk factor for postoperative infection after coronary artery bypass graft operation. *Journal of Thoracic and Cardiovascular Surgery* 1992;104(4):1092-1099.

Hébert PC, Schweitzer I, Calder L, et al. Review of the clinical practice literature on allogeneic red blood cell transfusion. *Can Med Assoc J* 1997;156:S9-S26

Nucci ML, Abuchowski A. The Search for Blood Substitutes. *Scientific American* February, 1998.

Goodnough LT, Brecher ME, Kanter MH, AuBuchon JP. Transfusion Medicine - Blood Transfusion. *N Engl J Med* 1999;340(6):445.

Goldman EB. Legal Considerations for Allogeneic Blood Transfusion. *Am J Surg* 1995;170(Suppl 6A):27S-31S.

Fisher F, Macdonald N, Sommerville A, et al., editors. *Medical Ethics Today: Its Practice and Philosophy,* from the British Medical Association's Ethics, Science and Information Division. London: BMJ Publishing Group; 1993.

Smallwood RA, Arnold P, Bastian H, et al. *General guidelines for medical practitioners on providing information to patients.* National Health and Medical Research Council. Commonwealth of Australia; 1993.

Riley GJ, Simmonds RL. Informed consent in modern medical practice. *Med J Aust* 1992;157:336-338.

Glorion B. The Medical Establishment and Bloodless Surgery: The View of the French Medical Council. In: Belghiti J, Castot M, Conseiller C, et al., editors. *Bloodless Surgery: Surgical and Anaesthetic Aspects; Legal and Ethical Issues.* Paris: Arnette Blackwell; 1997:143-146.

Chapter 5

(For chapters 5 & 6 also see references for Appendix Bloodless Medicine & Surgery Strategies)

Spence RK, Cernaianu AC, Carson J, et al. Transfusion and Surgery. *Curr Probl Surg* 1993;30(12):1103-1180.

Medical alternatives to blood transfusion. In: Huston P, editor. *Building a Blood System for the 21st Century. Proceedings and Recommendations.* Symposium on blood transfusion and the medical alternatives; 1997 Nov 3-4; Toronto, Canada. Ottawa: Health Canada (Canadian Federal Ministry of Health)/Canadian Blood Agency/Canadian Hemophilia Society; 1997.

Beris P. The Role of Iron in the Correction of Perioperative Anaemia. In: Belghiti J, Castot M, Conseiller C, et al., editors. *Bloodless Surgery: Surgical and Anaesthetic Aspects; Legal and Ethical Issues.* Paris: Arnette Blackwell; 1997:105-116.

Konrad Messmer on behalf of the Roundtable of Experts in Surgery Blood Management. Consensus Statement: Using Epoetin Alfa to Decrease the Risk of Allogeneic Blood Transfusion in the Surgical Setting. *Seminars in Hematology* 1996;33(2):78-80.

Canadian Orthopedic Perioperative Erythropoietin Study Group. Effectiveness of perioperative recombinant human erythropoietin in elective hip replacement. *Lancet* 1993;341:1227-1232.

Goldberg MA. Erythropoiesis, Erythropoietin, and Iron Metabolism in Elective Surgery: Preoperative Strategies for Avoiding Allogeneic Blood Exposure. *Am J Surg* 1995;170(suppl 6A):37S-43S.

Rutherford CJ, Schneider TJ, Dempsey H, et al. Efficacy of Different Dosing Regimens for Recombinant Human Erythropoietin in a Simulated Perisurgical Setting: The Importance of Iron Availability in Optimizing Response. *Am J Med* 1994;96:139-145.

Goldberg MA. Perioperative Epoetin Alfa Increases Red Blood Cell Mass and Reduces Exposure to Transfusions: Results of Randomized Clinical Trials. *Seminars in Hematology* 1997;34(3):41-47.

Brugnara C, Colella GM, Cremins J, et al. Effects of subcutaneous recombinant human erythropoietin in normal subjects: Development of decreased reticulocyte hemoglobin content and iron-deficient erythropoiesis. *J Lab Clin Med* 1994;123:660-667.

Horl WH, Cavill I, Macdougall IC, et al. Consensus Statement: How to diagnose and correct iron deficiency during r-huEPO therapy – a consensus report. *Nephrol Dial Transplant* 1996;11:246-250.

Borghi B, Fanelli G, Celleno D. Autotransfusion with predeposit-haemodilution and perioperative blood salvage: 20 years of experience. Rizzoli Study Group on Orthopaedic Anesthesia. *Int J Artif Organs* 1999;22(4):230-234.

Mercuriali F. Surgical procedures best suited to preoperative autologous blood donation. *Erythropoiesis: New Dimensions in the Treatment of Anaemia* 1997;8:16-25.

AuBuchon JP. Cost-effectiveness of Preoperative Autologous Blood Donation for Orthopedic and Cardiac Surgeries. *Am J Med* 1996;101(suppl 2A):38S-42S.

Blumberg N, Kirkely SA, Heal JM. A Cost Analysis of Autologous and Allogeneic Transfusions in Hip-Replacement Surgery. *Am J Surg* 1996;171:324-330.

Ovrum E, Holen EA, Tangen G, Oystese R. Cost savings with autotransfusion in connection with coronary surgery. *Tidsskr Nor Laegeforen* 1997;117(18):2616-2618.

Price TH, Goodnough LT, Vogler WR, et al. The effect of recombinant human erythropoietin on the efficacy of autologous blood donation in patients with low hematocrits: a multicenter, randomized, double-blind, controlled trial. *Transfusion* 1996;36:29-36.

Spence RK. Emerging Trends in Surgical Blood Transfusion. *Seminars in Hematology* 1997;34(3):48-53.

Gombotz H, Metzler H, List WF. Methods for reduction of perioperative bleeding. *Br J Anaesth* 1998;81(suppl 1):62-66.

Atabek U, Alvarez R, Pello M, et al. Erythropoeitin Accelerates Hematocrit Recovery in Post-Surgical Anemia. *Am Surg* 1995;61:74-77

Wolff M, Fandrey J, Hirner A, et al. Perioperative use of recombinant human erythropoietin in patients refusing blood transfusions. Pathophysiological considerations based on 5 cases. *Eu J Haematol* 1997;58:154-159.

Macdougall IC, Hutton RD, Cavill I, et al. Poor response to treatment of renal anaemia with erythropoietin corrected by iron given intravenously. *Br Med J* 1989;299:157-158.

Hoigne R, Breymann C, Kunzi UP, Brunner F. Parenteral iron therapy: problems and possible solutions. *Schweiz Med Wochenschr* 1998;128(14):528-535.

Dudrick SJ, O'Donnell JJ, Raleigh DP, et al. Rapid Restoration of Red Blood Cell Mass in Severely Anemic Surgical Patients Who Refuse Transfusion. *Arch Surg* 1985;120:721-727.

Van Iperen CE, Biesma DH, Van De Wiel A, Marx JJM. Erythropoietic response to acute and chronic anaemia: focus on postoperative anaemia. *Br J Anaesth* 1998;81(suppl 1):2-5.

Adamson JW. Regulation of Red Blood Cell Production. *Am J Med* 1996;101(suppl 2A):4S-6S.

Koury MJ. Investigating Erythropoietin Resistance. *N Engl J Med* 1993;328(3):205-206.

Chernow B, Salem M, Stacey J. Blood conservation – A critical care imperative. *Critical Care Medicine* 1991;19(3):313-314.

Smoller BR, Kruskall MS. Phlebotomy for Diagnostic Laboratory Tests in Adults: Pattern of Use and Effect on Transfusion Requirements. *N Engl J Med* 1986;314:1233-1235.

Silverberg DS, Blum M, Peer G, et al. Intravenous Ferric Saccharate as an Iron Supplement in Dialysis Patients. *Nephron* 1996;72:413-417.

Bennett DR, Shulman IA. Practical issues when confronting the patient who refuses blood transfusion therapy. *Am J Clin Pathol* 1997;107(suppl 1):S23-S27.

Meletis J, Smarkos M, Michali E, et al. Correction of anaemia and thrombocytopenia in a case of adult Type I osteopetrosis with recombinant human erythropoietin (rHuEPO). *British Journal of Haematology* 1995;89:911-913.

Krantz SB. Erythropoietin. *Blood* 1991;77:419-434.

Dessypris EN, Graber SE, Krantz SB, Stone WJ. Effects of Recombinant Erythropoietin on the Concentration and Cycling Status of Human Marrow Hematopoietic Progenitor Cells In Vivo. *Blood* 1988;72(6):2060-2062.

Stehling L, Zauder HL. How low can we go? Is there a way to know? *Transfusion* 1990;30(1):1-3.

Allen JB, Allen FB. The Minimum Acceptable Level of Hemoglobin. *International Anesthesiology Clinics* 1982;20(4):1-22.

Stowell C. When to Pull the Trigger – Making the Decision To Transfuse Red Blood Cells. *Laboratory Medicine* 1995;26(1):55-62.

Weiskopf RB, Viele MK, Feiner J, et al. Human Cardiovascular and Metabolic Response to Acute, Severe Isovolemic Anemia. *JAMA* 1998;279(3):217-221.

Lieberman JA, Weiskopf RB, Kelley SD et al. Critical Oxygen Delivery in Conscious Humans is Less Than 7.3 ml $O_2 \cdot kg^{-1} \cdot min^{-1}$. *Anesthesiology* 2000; 92:407-413.

Van Woerkens ECSM, Trouwborst A, van Lanschot JJB. Profound Hemodilution: What Is the Critical Level of Hemodilution at Which Oxygen Delivery-Dependent Oxygen Consumption Starts in an Anesthetized Human? *Anesth Analg* 1992;75:818-821.

Greenburg AG. A Physiologic Basis for Red Blood Cell Transfusion Decisions. *Am J Surg* 1995;107(suppl 6A):44S-48S.

Greenburg AG. Pathophysiology of Anemia. *Am J Med* 1996;101(suppl 1):7S-11S.

Spence RK. Anemia in the patient undergoing surgery and the decision to transfuse. A review. *Clin Orthop* 1998;357:19-29.

Chen AY, Carson JL. Perioperative management of anaemia. *Br J Anaesth* 1998;81(suppl 1):20-24.

Carson JL, Chen AY. In search of the transfusion trigger. *Clin Orthop* 1998;357:30-35.

Bracey AW, Radovancevic R, Riggs SA, et al. Lowering the hemoglobin threshold for transfusion in coronary artery bypass procedures: effect on patient outcome. *Transfusion* 1999;39(10):1070-1077.

Viele MK, Weiskopf RB. What can we learn about the need for transfusion from patients who refuse blood? The experience with Jehovah's Witnesses. *Transfusion* 1994;34(5):396-401.

Saxen S, Rabinowitz AP, Johnson C, Shulman IA. Iron-Deficiency Anemia: A Medically Treatable Chronic Anemia as a Model for Transfusion Overuse. *Am J Med* 1993;94:120-124.

Salem MR, Manley S, Crystal GJ, Heyman HJ. Perioperative Hemoglobin Requirements. In: Salem MR, editor. *Blood Conservation in the Surgical Patient.* Baltimore: Williams & Wilkins 1996: 107-145.

Brimacombe J, Skippen P, Talbutt P. Acute Anaemia to a Haemoglobin of 14 g/L with Survival. *Anaesthesia and Intensive Care* 1991;19(4):581-583.

Akingbola OA, Custer JR, Bunchman TE, et al. Management of severe anemia without transfusion in a pediatric Jehovah's Witness patient. *Critical Care Medicine* 1994;22(3):524-528.

Mann MC, Votto J, Kambe J, McNamee MJ. Management of the Severely Anemic Patient Who Refuses Transfusion: Lessons Learned during the Care of a Jehovah's Witness. *Ann*

Intern Med 1992;117:1042-1048.

Kitchens CS. Are Transfusions Overrated? Surgical Outcome of Jehovah's Witnesses. *Am J Med* 1993;94:117-119.

Nearman HS, Eckhauser ML. Postoperative management of a severely anemic Jehovah's Witness. *Critical Care Medicine* 1983;11(2):142-143.

Howell PJ, Bamber PA. Severe acute anaemia in a Jehovah's Witness. 1987;42:44-48.

Neff TA, Stocker R, Wight E, Spahn DR. Extreme Intraoperative Blood Loss and Hemodilution in a Jehovah's Witness: New Aspects in Postoperative Management. *Anesthesiology* 1999;91:1949-1951.

Spence RK, Carson JA, Poses R, et al. Elective Surgery without Transfusion: Influence of Preoperative Hemoglobin Level and Blood Loss on Mortality. *Am J Surg* 1990;159:320-324.

Langone J. Bloodless Surgery. In: *Time*. Special Issue: Heroes of Medicine. 1997.

Chapter 6

Han FFY, Iron Therapy – Choice of agents. *Bloodless Surgery Update* 1998;3(1):3-4.

Hardman J. *Goodman and Gilman's: The Pharmacological Basis of Therapeutics,* 9th ed. New York: McGraw Hill; 1996.

Smith AG. Prescribing iron. *Prescriber's J* 1997;37(2):82-87.

Laurence DR, Bennett PN. *Clinical pharmacology,* 7th ed. Edinburgh: Churchill Livingstone; 1992.

Erber W. Management of iron deficiency. *Royal Perth Hospital Drug Bulletin* Sept-Oct 1993;3(5).

Crystal FJ, Salem MR. Acute Normovolemic Hemodilution. In: Salem MR, editor. *Blood Conservation in the Surgical Patient.* Baltimore: Williams & Wilkins; 1996:168-187.

Monk TG, Goodnough LT, Brecher ME, et al. Acute normovolemic hemodilution can replace preoperative autologous blood donation as a standard of care for autologous blood procurement in radical prostatectomy. *Anesth Analg* 1997:85:953-958.

Rottman G, Ness PM. Acute normovolemic hemodilution is a legitimate alternative to allogeneic blood transfusion. *Transfusion* 1998;38:477-480.

Goodnough LT. Acute Normovolemic Hemodilution. *Transfusion Alternatives in Transfusion Medicine* 1999;1(1):12-16.

Stehling L, Zauder HL. Acute normovolemic hemodilution. *Transfusion* 1991;31(9):857-868.

Monk TG, Goodnough LT. Acute Normovolemic Hemodilution. *Clinical Orthopaedics and Related Research* 1998;357:74-81.

Monk TG, Goodnough LT, Brecher ME, et al. A Prospective Randomized Comparison of Three Blood Conservation Strategies for Radical Prostatectomy. *Anesthesiology* 1999;91(1):24-33.

Kochntop DE, Belani KG. Acute Severe Hemodilution to a Hemoglobin of 1.3 g/dL Tolerated in the Presence of Mild Hypothermia. *Anesthesiology* 1999;90(6):1798-1799.

Crystal FJ, Salem MR, Principles of Oxygen Transport. In: Salem MR, editor. *Blood Conservation in the Surgical Patient.* Baltimore: Williams & Wilkins; 1996:79-91.

Goodnough LT, Monk TG, Brecher ME. Autologous blood procurement in the surgical setting: lessons learned in the last 10 years. *Vox Sang* 1996;71:133-141.

Royal College of Physicians of Edinburgh Consensus Conference on Autologous Transfusion November 1998. Desmond M, et al. Perioperative red cell salvage: a case for implementing the 1995 consensus statement. *Transfusion Medicine* 1999;9:265-268.

Gombotz H, Kulier A. Intraoperative Autotransfusion of RBC and PRP. *Transfusion Alternatives in Transfusion Medicine* 1999;1(3):5-13.

Tawes RL Jr., ed. *Autotransfusion: Therapeutic Principles and Trends.* Detroit: Gregory Appleton; 1997.

Salem MR, Manley S. Blood Conservation Techniques. In: Salem MR, editor. *Blood Conservation in the Surgical Patient.* Baltimore: Williams & Wilkins; 1996:92-106.

Griffel MI, Kaufman BS. Pharmacology of Colloids and Crystalloids. *Critical Care Clinics* 1992;8(2):235-253.

Haljamäe H. Use of fluids in trauma. *International Journal of Intensive Care* 1999:20-29.

Boerema I, Meyne NG, Brummelkamp WK, et al. Life without blood: a study of the influence of high atmospheric pressure and hypothermia on dilution of blood. *J Cardiovasc Surg* 1960;1:133-146.

Kindwall EP, Goldman RW, editors. Anemia, Exceptional Blood Loss. In: *Hyperbaric Medical Procedures.* Milwaukee, Wis: Saint Lukes Medical Center; 1988:28-29.

Myking O, Schreiner A. Hyperbaric Oxygen in Hemolytic Crisis. *JAMA* 1974;227(10):1161-1162.

McLoughlin PL, Cope TM, Harrison JC. Hyperbaric oxygen therapy in the management of severe acute anaemia in a Jehovah's Witness. *Anaesthesia* 1999;54:879-898.

Leach RM, Rees PJ, Wilmshurst P. Clinical review. *ABC of oxygen* -Hyperbaric oxygen therapy. *Br Med J* 1998;317:1140-1143.

Tibbles PM, Edelsberg JS. Hyperbaric-Oxygen Therapy. *N Engl J Med* 1996;334(25):1642-1648.

Erber WN, Tan J, Grey D, Lown JAG. Use of unrefrigerated fresh whole blood in massive transfusion. *Med J Aust* 1996;15:11-13.

Mattox KL, Mattox KL, Brundage SI, Hirshberg A. Initial resuscitation. *New Horizons* 1999;7:4-9.

Mattox KL. Introducttion, background, and future projections of damage control surgery. *Surg Clin North Am* 1997;77(4):753-759.

Bickell WH, Wall MJ, Pepe PE, et al. Immediate versus Delayed Fluid Resuscitation for Hypotensive Patients With Penetrating Torso Injuries. *N Engl J Med* 1994;331(17):1105-1109.

Wall MJ, Granchi T, Liscum K, Aucar J, Mattox KL. Delayed versus immediate fluid resuscitation in patients with penetrating trauma: subgroup analysis. *J Trauma* 1995;39(1):173.

Richardson JD, Polk HC. Reoperation for Trauma. *Ann Surg* 1995;222(1):1-2.

Hirshberg A, Mattox KL. Planned Reoperation for Severe Trauma. *Ann Surg* 1995;222(1):3-8.

Rotondo MF, Schwab CW, McGonigal MD, Phillips GR 3rd, Fruchterman TM, et al. 'Damage Control': An Approach for Improved Survival in Exsanguinating Penetrating Abdominal Injury. *J Trauma* 1993;35(3):375-383.

Gombotz H, Metzler H, List WF. Methods for reduction of perioperative bleeding. *Br J Anaesth* 1998;81(Suppl 1):62-66.

Spahn DR. Benefits of Red Blood Cell Transfusion: Where is the Evidence? *Transfusion Alternatives in Transfusion Medicine* 1999;1(1):6-10.

Weiskopf RB. Do we know when to transfuse red cells to treat acute anemia? *Transfusion* 1998;38:517-521.

Chapter 7

Chen AY, Carson JL. Perioperative management of anaemia. *Br J Anaesth* 1998;81(suppl 1):20-24.

Carson JL, Duff A, Berlin JA, et al. Perioperative Blood Transfusion and Postoperative Mortality. *JAMA* 1998;279(3):199-205.

Hardy JF, Martineau R, Couturier A, et al. Influence of haemoglobin concentration after extracorporeal circulation on mortality and morbidity in patients undergoing cardiac surgery. *Br J Anaesth* 1998;81(suppl 1):38-45.

Spence RK. Preoperative packed cell volume necessary for patients undergoing elective surgery. *Br J Anaesth* 1998;81(suppl 1):50-55.

Hébert PC, For the Transfusion Requirements in Critical Care Investigators and the Canadian Critical Care Trials Group. Transfusion requirements in critical care (TRICC): a multicentre, randomized, controlled clinical study. *Br J Anaesth* 1998;81(suppl 1):25-33.

Marik PE, Sibbald WJ. Effect of stored-blood transfusion on oxgen delivery in patients with sepsis. *JAMA* 1993;269(23):3024-3029.

Fitzgerald RD, Martin CM, Dietz GE, et al. Transfusing red blood cells stored in citrate phosphate dextrose adenine-1 for 28 days fails to improve tissue oxygenation in rats. *Crit Care Med* 1997;25(5):726-732.

Corwin HL. Blood Transfusion: First Do No Harm! *Chest* 1999;116:1149-1150.

Dunphy JE. Ethics in Surgery: Going Beyond Good Science. *Bulletin* 1978;63(6).

Spahn DR. Benefits of Red Blood Cell Transfusion: Where is the Evidence?" *Transfusion Alternatives in Transfusion Medicine* 1999;1(1):6-10.

Weiskopf RB. More on the Changing Indications for Transfusion of Blood and Blood Components during Anesthesia. *Anesthesiology* 1996;84(3):498-501.

Spahn DR, van Brempt R, Theilmeier G, et al. Perflubron emulsion delays blood transfusions in orthopedic surgery. European Perflubron Emulsion Study Group. *Anesthesiology* 1999;91(5):1195-1208.

Habler O, Kleen M, Messmer K. Artificial oxygen carriers: Alternatives to homologous blood transfusion? *Zentralbl Chir* 1999;124(4):260-270.

Lamy M, Remy B, Deby-Dupont G. Modified Haemoglobins and Perfluorocarbons as Oxygen-Carrying Solutions: Characteristics and Possible Applications. In: Belghiti J, Castot M, Conseiller C, et al., editors. *Bloodless Surgery: Surgical and Anaesthetic Aspects; Legal and Ethical Issues.* Paris: Arnette Blackwell; 1997:117-129.

Baron JF. Haemoglobin therapy in clinical practice: use and characteristics of DCLHb. *Br J Anaesth* 1998;81(suppl 1):34-37.

Medical alternatives to blood transfusion. In: Huston P, editor. *Building a Blood System for the 21st Century. Proceedings and Recommendations.* Symposium on blood transfusion and the medical alternatives; 1997 Nov 3-4; Toronto, Canada. Ottawa: Health Canada (Canadian Federal Ministry of Health)/Canadian Blood Agency/Canadian Hemophilia Society; 1997. p. 57-88.

Prowse CV. Alternatives to standard blood transfusion: availability and promise. *Transfusion Medicine* 1999;9:287-299.

Robb N. Concerns of Patients, MDs are Transforming Transfusion Medicine. *Can Med Assoc J* 1996;154(3):391-396.

Tough B. The Legal Implications of the New Blood System for Health Care Providers and Governments. In: Huston P, editor. *Building a Blood System for the 21st Century. Proceedings and Recommendations.* Symposium on blood transfusion and the medical alternatives; 1997 Nov 3-4; Toronto, Canada. Ottawa: Health Canada/Canadian Blood Agency/Canadian Hemophilia Society; 1997:33-34.

Levinson RK. Bloodless surgery. *N J Med* 1999;96(8):39-41.

Farmer SL. What is bloodless surgery? *Bloodless Surgery Bulletin* 1998;2(1):1-2.

Vernon S, Pfeifer GM. Are You Ready for Bloodless Surgery? *American Journal of Nursing* 1997;97(9):40-46.

Maness CP, Russell SM, Altonji P, Allmendinger P. Bloodless Medicine and Surgery. *AORNJ* 1998;67:144-152.

Ward WF. The development of a hospital-based bloodless surgery protocol. *Erythropoiesis: New Dimensions in the Treatment of Anaemia* 1998;8:102-111.

Salem-Schatz SR, Avorn J, Soumerai SB. Influence of Clinical Knowledge, Organizational Context, and Practice Style on Transfusion Decision Making: Implications for Practice Change Strategies. *JAMA* 1990;264(4):476-483.

British Committee for Standards in Haematology, Blood Transfusion Task Force in collaboration with the Royal College of Nursing and the Royal College of Surgeons of England. The administration of blood and blood components and the management of transfused patients. *Transfusion Medicine* 1999;9:227-238.

Rosencrantz D, Shander A, Ozawa S, Spence R. Establishing a Bloodless Medicine and Surgery Center. In: Stehling L, Spence R, Contreras M, et al, editors. *Transfusion Medicine and Alternatives to Blood Transfusion.* Paris: R & J Éditions Médicales; 2000:511-516.

....THE CONTINUING STORY

If you need to keep abreast of the fast evolving bloodless medicine and surgery scene, Media Masters, publishers of *Your Body, Your Choice*, have established a special database to meet your requirements. The authors and publishers are continuing to monitor and document this stunning healthcare revolution that has such massive long-term implications for both medicine and mankind.

As dictated by scientific and medical breakthroughs, there will be updated editions of *Your Body, Your Choice*. Furthermore, depending on the manner and timing of these advances, separate bulletins, complementary to existing chapters and topics in the main body of the book, will be made available. To ensure you are kept informed, please signal your interest to Media Masters.

You can contact us through our direct email addresses:
In Singapore: medmas@mbox3.singnet.com.sg
In Australia: mediam@bigpond.com
Alternatively, you can visit Media Masters website at:
www.mediamasters.com.sg

To further assist you, here is a list of our main distributors outside North America:

United Kingdom & Europe
John Wilson Booksales,
1 High Street, Princes Risborough,
Buckinghamshire HP27 0AG, UK.
Tel: (01844) 275 927, Fax: (01844) 274 402
Email: jw@jwbs.co.uk

Australia
Capricorn Link,
Unit 2/13 Carrington Road,
Castle Hill, NSW 2154
Tel: (02) 9899 8322, Fax: (02) 9899 8221
Email: caplink@eisa.net.au

New Zealand
Shandwick (NZ),
2 Woodward Street,
Wellington 6015
Tel: (04) 472 4190, Fax: (04) 471 2278
Email: execsec@shandwick.co.nz

Singapore
STP Distributors Pte Ltd,
Pasir Panjang Districentre,
Block 1, #03-01A Pasir Panjang Road, Singapore 118480
Tel: 276 7626, Fax: 276 7119
Email: stpbk@corp.tpl.com.sg

Malaysia
STP Distributors (M) Sdn Bhd,
Lot 46, Subang Hi-Tech Industrial Park
Batu Tiga, 40000 Shah Alam, Selangor, Darul Ehsan
Tel: (03) 735 1511, Fax: (03) 736 4620
Email: ivan@tpg.com.my

Philippines
National Book Store,
125 Pioneer Street, Mandaluyong City,
Philippines.
Tel: (02) 631 3061 to 66, Fax: (02) 634 0376
Email: purchbooks@nationalbookstore.com.ph

India
The Variety Book Depot,
A.V.G.Bhawan, M-3 Connaught Circus,
New Delhi – 110 001
Tel: (011) 332 7175, Fax: (011) 371 4335
Email: variety@nde.vsnl.net.in

ACKNOWLEDGEMENTS

Operating Room Photography:
Good Samaritan Hospital, Los Angeles, USA, and Fremantle Kaleeya Hospital, Western Australia.

Front Cover:
Peter Goodall

Other pictures:
Conmed Corporation and Stubber Medical (photo of Argon Beam Coagulator). Jan Graziani and Center for Bloodless Medicine and Surgery, Our Lady of Resurrection Hospital, Chicago Ill. (photos of patient in single hyperbaric chamber and hospital facade). Community Memorial Hospital, Ventura, CA, (photos illustrating "How to Access Bloodless Surgery"). Alliance Pharmaceutical Corp. (photo of Oxygent ™). Computer Motion (photo of robotic surgery by Bobbi Bennett © 1999). The Western Australian Centre for Pathology and Medical Research (photos of blood storage). Kenneth Wagner (Photography at Good Samaritan Hospital, Los Angeles).

Color diagrams:
Karen Briedums

Black and white diagrams:
Demetrio Miraflor

Reviewers:

Dr Richard Spence	(USA)
Dr Aryeh Shander	(USA)
Dr Manuel Estioko	(USA)
Mr Jan Wade	(USA)
Mr Peter Earnshaw	(United Kingdom)
Dr Wendy Erber	(Australia)
Dr Vladimir Martyn	(Australia)
Dr Simon Towler	(Australia)
Dr Michael Wren	(Australia)
Dr Julie McMorrow	(Australia)
Mr Zenon Bodnaruk	(Canada)
Dr James Kong	(Hong Kong)

ABOUT THE AUTHORS

SHANNON FARMER is Coordinator of the Center for Bloodless Medicine and Surgery at Fremantle Kaleeya Hospital in Western Australia. As coordinator, he liaises with patients, reviews policies and procedures for the center and develops education programs for hospital staff, doctors and the community. Farmer is the chairperson of his hospital's bloodless medicine and surgery advisory committee and also works as a consultant in these specialties for a number of leading health groups. At the same time he is heavily involved in data collection and medical research analysis and is called upon frequently to lecture on these subjects.

Farmer was involved in setting up Kaleeya's bloodless surgery program in 1990, the first private hospital in Australia to establish such a center. The program has since broadened to include specialists in other hospitals in the city. After acquiring a deep interest in the practice following a study tour of bloodless surgery centers in the United States, Farmer has become one of the more knowledgeable people on the subject. He travels widely to attend international seminars and is a member of the National Association for Bloodless Medicine and Surgery (NABMS). NABMS is part of a worldwide network linking coordinators, researchers and some of the world's leading surgeons and medical specialists. Farmer is also a member of the Network for Advancement of Transfusion Alternatives (NATA), comprising world renowned experts in the field of blood conservation. NATA was founded in Graz, Austria, to disseminate medical and scientific information about transfusion medicine and alternatives.

DAVID WEBB is a journalist and former metropolitan newspaper editor whose interest in bloodless medicine and surgery began during his activities as a consultant with Fremantle Kaleeya Hospital. Webb's increasing understanding of bloodless surgery and realization of its vital importance for health care prompted a joint decision with Farmer to write this book. The outcome is this fascinating exploration of a subject with massive implications for the world health scene. That it is the first time a book has ever been written on these matters for the lay person says much for the co-authors' two-profession fusion of expertise and editorial experience.

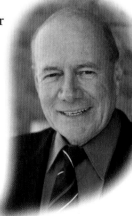

NOTES

NOTES